*Yum*Universe
Pantry
<u>TO</u> Plate

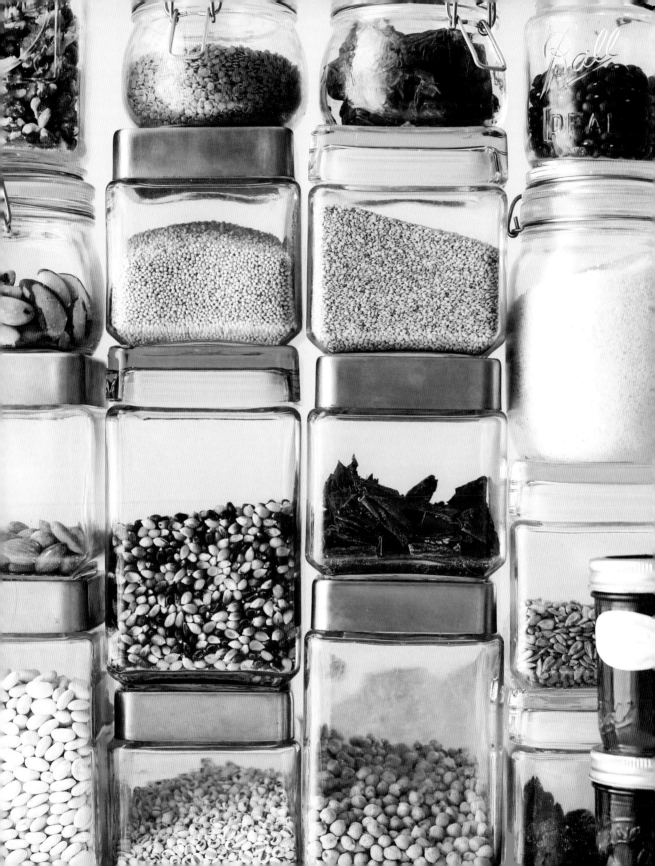

*Yum*Universe
Pantry
<u>to</u> Plate

Improvise Meals You Love—
from What You Have!

Heather Crosby
Author of *YumUniverse*

THE EXPERIMENT

NEW YORK

YᴜᴍUɴɪᴠᴇʀsᴇ Pᴀɴᴛʀʏ ᴛᴏ Pʟᴀᴛᴇ: *Improvise Meals You Love—from What You Have!*

Copyright © 2017 by Heather Crosby
Illustrations and photographs copyright © 2017 by Heather Crosby with the exception of:
Photographs on pages v, viii, 13, 29, 309 bottom left, and 310 © Pang Tubhirun
Photographs on pages 7, 306 top right, 307 middle right, 308 top left, and 312 © Marta Sasinowska

The Experiment, LLC
220 East 23rd Street, Suite 301
New York, NY 10010-4674
theexperimentpublishing.com

This book contains the opinions and ideas of its author. It is intended to provide helpful and informative material on the subjects addressed in the book. It is sold with the understanding that the author and publisher are not engaged in rendering medical, health, or any other kind of personal professional services in the book. The author and publisher specifically disclaim all responsibility for any liability, loss, or risk—personal or otherwise—that is incurred as a consequence, directly or indirectly, of the use and application of any of the contents of this book.

Many of the designations used by manufacturers and sellers to distinguish their products are claimed as trademarks. Where those designations appear in this book and The Experiment was aware of a trademark claim, the designations have been capitalized.

The Experiment's books are available at special discounts when purchased in bulk for premiums and sales promotions as well as for fund-raising or educational use. For details, contact us at info@theexperimentpublishing.com.

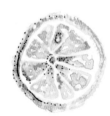

Library of Congress Cataloging-in-Publication Data

Names: Crosby, Heather, author.
Title: YumUniverse pantry to plate : improvise meals you love--from what you
    have!--plant-packed, gluten-free, your way! / by Heather Crosby.
Other titles: Pantry to plate
Description: New York, NY : Experiment, LLC, [2017] | Includes index.
Identifiers: LCCN 2016048074| ISBN 9781615193400 (pbk.) | ISBN 9781615193417
    (ebook)
Subjects: LCSH: Natural foods--Health aspects. | Cooking (Natural foods) |
    Vegetarian cooking. | Gluten-free diet--Recipes. | LCGFT: Cookbooks.
Classification: LCC RM237.55 .C764 2017 | DDC 641.5/636--dc23
LC record available at https://lccn.loc.gov/2016048074

ISBN 978-1-61519-340-0
Ebook ISBN 978-1-61519-341-7

Cover, illustrations, and text design by Heather Crosby
Cover photograph by Heather Crosby
Author photographs by Pang Tubhirun

Manufactured in China
Distributed by Workman Publishing Company, Inc.
Distributed simultaneously in Canada by Thomas Allen & Son Ltd.

First printing May 2017
10 9 8 7 6 5 4 3 2 1

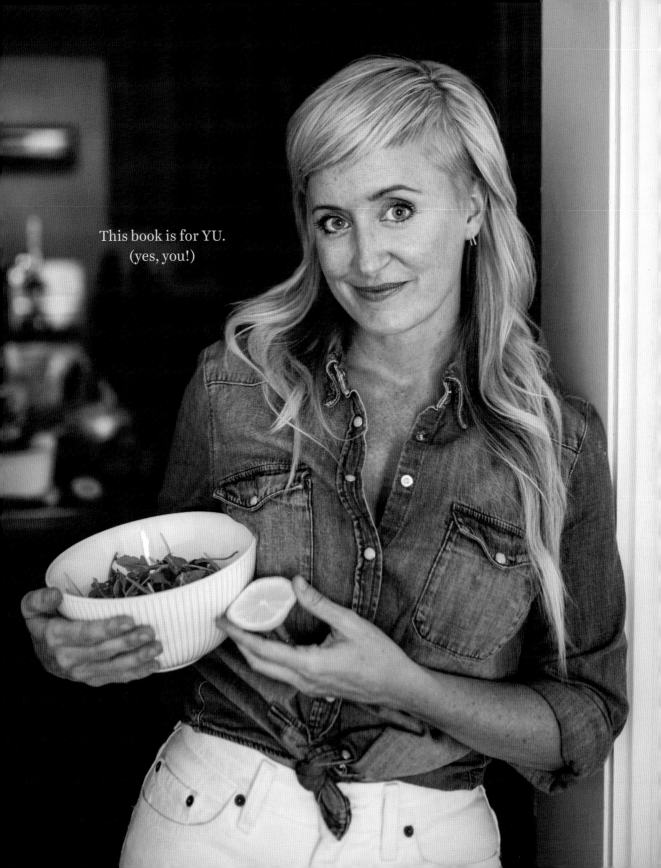

This book is for YU.
(yes, you!)

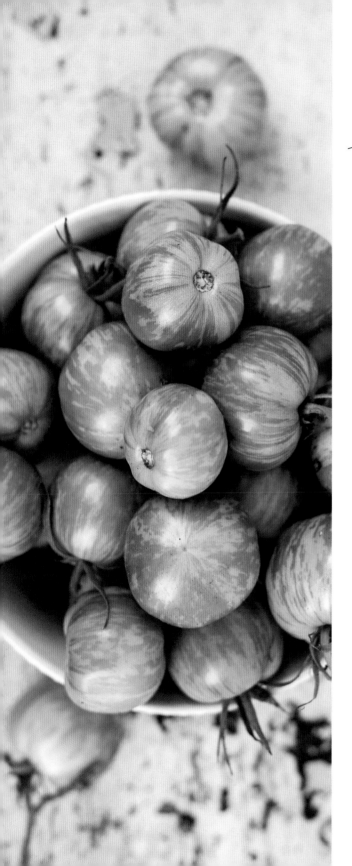

Contents

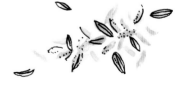

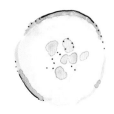

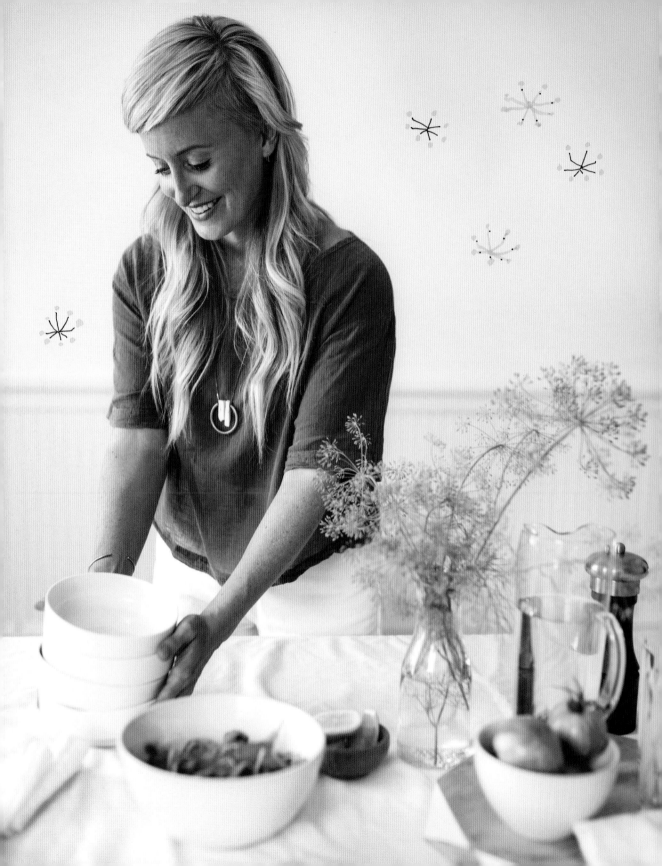

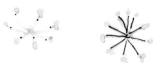

Hello, from a Former Veggie Phobe

I was raised on comfort food and sweets—it's in my DNA, and in the bedrock of my memories and traditions. For most of my life, I avoided vegetables of any kind (except white potatoes) and it wasn't until I got sick in my early twenties and was told "meds for the rest of your life" that I decided something had to change—my terrible diet was a good place to start. I had to be able to enjoy delicious food without compromising my health, but I had no clue how it was done.

At that time, I assumed "healthy" foods were bland, boring, a hassle, and pricey. But since I wasn't familiar with whole food ingredients, that meant that I had no real "rules" for how they should be prepared and incorporated into meals—I had free rein. So, I freestyled—making changes I could manage and be excited about. Eventually, small daily efforts compounded and became health-boosting habits. By finding delicious whole food substitutions for my comfort-food faves, I realized that smart choices and tasty choices don't have to be mutually exclusive.

Cashews are buttery and creamy. Can they be blended to make a velvety, cheese-like cream sauce? Yes. Cooked buckwheat is similar to the texture of the sausage patties my grandfather used to make—perfect for veggie burgers. In this book, you'll find a version of my grandmother Maudie's tomato sauce, sans bacon but with all the smoky flavor. See, I know you have tradition and memory attached to food, too. And we don't have to say goodbye to these important parts of life for health's sake. It's a miracle (just ask my mother), but I love vegetables now, and I want to show you how versatile, delicious, and freeing they can be.

Hearts,
Heather

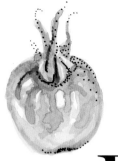

Pantry-to-Plate Cooking

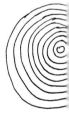

Fact: I'm no good at following recipes. This gal needs freedom to play, change her mind, explore, color outside of the lines, and make it up as she goes along. I didn't realize that this was actually my real-time approach to cooking until I heard myself answering questions like "How do you cook for yourself on a daily basis?" with "A lot of the time I just throw a bunch of colorful ingredients into a skillet, season to taste, and I'm done." Boring? Maybe. But real? Definitely. A lot of the time, meals in my home are created using a "template" I've committed to memory, then I change the players based on everything from my food mood to what's in season to what I simply have in the pantry, fridge, or garden. I don't think I'm alone here—many people cook without a recipe on a day-to-day basis. We're a busy lot.

Now, with that said, many folks also cook using recipes, too! Recipes show us what's possible, they give us structure when we want to follow instead of lead, they introduce us to new techniques and tastes, and they reward us for our efforts with each tasty bite. Recipe cooking requires us to shop, prepare, slow down, spend the time. It's a special practice because we've been inspired by something we want to try, and to try is to grow. A recipe is designed to be shared—the developer of that recipe put love and care into it, no doubt thinking of a happy eater enjoying it at some point. It's a beautiful ripple effect.

This book provides the tools for *both* approaches to cooking because sometimes we're prepared for a recipe, and sometimes not so much. Sometimes we love the look of a recipe, and sometimes there's one pesky ingredient that keeps us from giving it a go. Sometimes mealtime arrives and we don't have a clue what we're going to cook. And if we do, we may not have all of the fixings, or we're not up for anything super involved. Sometimes we have a fridge full of vegetables that we aren't

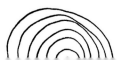

used to using, or there's just too much of it to use before it goes bad. Maybe we have a mixed-diet table to feed, or we had a grand plan to make a new Mexican recipe on Wednesday, but that day arrives and we've changed our mind—we want Italian. No, Indian.

This is life. And *Pantry to Plate* is an approach you can return to again and again for countless impromptu and customized meals. Reclaim the freedom to make it up as you go along and build confidence to "wing it" in the kitchen—without compromising your health.

In these pages, you'll find thirty templates to mix and match and create meals you love. From those thirty series of steps, almost 100 recipes have been developed to show you what's possible using those simple guidelines. You can follow a recipe to the letter, or you can riff off of the template it came from to make it your own—there are infinite possibilities—YumUniverse style.

Pantry-to-plate cooking provides myriad choices for those who want them, inspiration for those who need some, and boundaries for those who find comfort from them. This is your playbook—write down what you create, dog-ear the pages, give it some colorful character with a spill or splatter.

Healthful meal preparation isn't about deprivation, spending excessive time, or pricey ingredients—it's about making it work. So, go ahead and buy the wacky-looking heirloom veggies from the farmers' market, and use last night's tacos to make a breakfast scramble, wrap, or soup. With the tools in this book, meal creation begins from where you are, with what you have, right now.

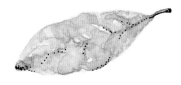

Your Very Own Recipe Playbook

This book is organized by meals we love to eat, but the templates will work whenever. Nothing taps into childhood feel-good feels like waffles for dinner, right? So you can make the rules; there is one master template for on-the-fly pantry-to-plate creations, followed by recipes that are inspired by that template. We're celebrating a keeping-it-real approach to cooking here that takes the pressure off being "healthy" and ultimately adds more color, fun, and flavor to our life. And by "life" I mean the long haul and overall health and well-being.

NO JUDGMENTS

The creations in this book happen to be gluten-free and veg-inspired because I love the variety these foods bring to my menu rotation, the flavors they've introduced to my taste buds, and the healing they've helped me achieve. But this book is for anyone who simply wants to eat more clean, whole foods. I'm not here to judge or tell you how to live your life. I'm here to share what's possible.

If you eat animal or gluten-containing products, these ingredients can easily be added to the templates and recipes in this book. Let's just move veggies from the side of the plate to the center while you're here.

PLANNING FOR BUSY PEOPLE

Planning doesn't have to mean writing up meal plans, organizing shopping lists, or collecting recipes. It can be as simple as soaking some grains while you sleep, freezing leftover soup into flavor cubes, or doubling the batch of pancakes you made Sunday morning to freeze for popping in the toaster throughout the week. If we just squeak out a bit of forethought, we set ourselves up for smart choices. Keep the pantry stocked, fresh aromatics like onions and garlic on hand, and prepared ingredients like beans and grains in the fridge, but don't overthink it.

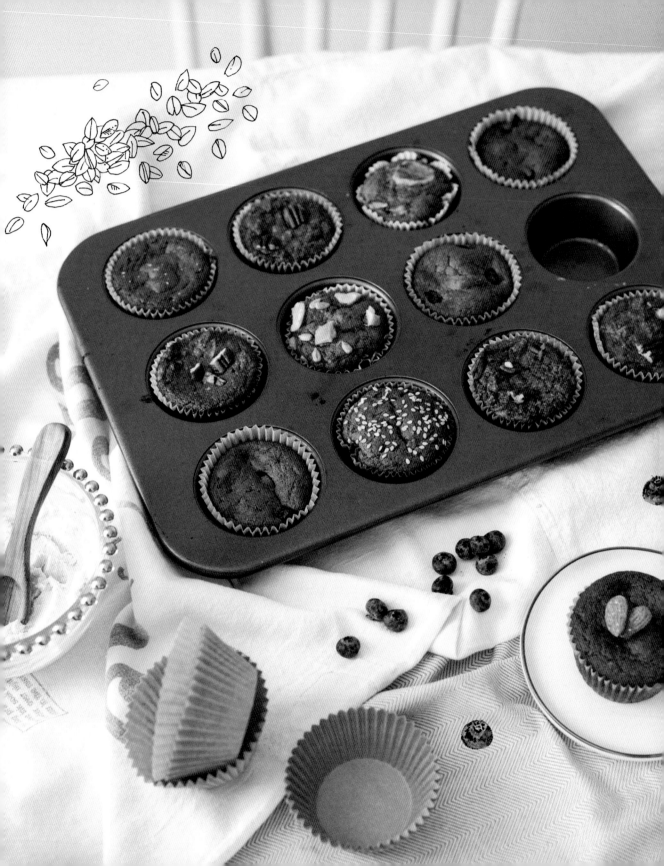

Tips & Tricks

ADD MORE GOOD STUFF TO THE ROUTINE

We don't grow unless we go outside of our comfort zone, but taking on too much at once can lead to resentment and/or burnout. Keep it simple—make one new recipe, or try one new template per week.

KEEP IT REAL

Use clean, whole food, fresh ingredients whenever possible for the best flavor and nutrition. I'll always call for soaked, fresh-cooked legumes and beans, but you can definitely use canned.

I also prefer using fresh herbs and goodies like ginger, but you can use dried if that's easier for you. Typically, dried herbs and spices are three times more concentrated than fresh. For example, if a template or recipe calls for 1 tablespoon of fresh herbs, you need only 1 teaspoon of dried. Check out the measurement-conversion reference on page 297.

Whenever I call for bases like Cream Cheese (page 128), Coconut Yogurt (page 94), or any sauces like BBQ (page 30), know that you can use store-bought items instead of homemade—just keep it clean. No unpronounceable ingredients and/or added sugar.

READ, THEN COOK

Please read the entire template or recipe at least once before you begin cooking. Some steps are time sensitive and require you to act quickly or plan ahead.

THINK OUTSIDE THE BOX

One morning's scramble leftovers can become another night's tacos. Repurpose ingredients and leftovers so cooking is freedom instead of a chore. Spin what you already like in a new way. Example: If you love a cup of Earl Grey tea with honey and cream, use that flavor combo to make Granola (page 45) with Almond Milk (page 101).

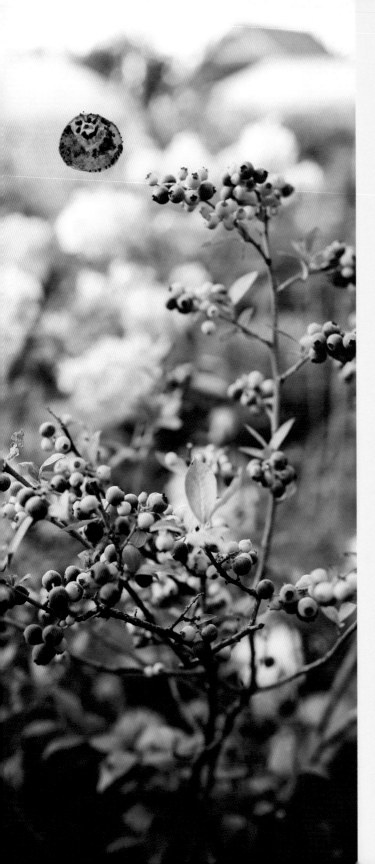

YOU DO YOU

If you're not plant-based or gluten-free, other ingredients can easily be added to the templates and recipes in this book. They're designed to be a springboard for your own creations.

A few quick thoughts:

Gluten-Free, Soy-Free

If you have a gluten sensitivity or celiac disease, it's important to buy ingredients labeled "gluten-free," as the FDA only allows packaged foods with less than 20 ppm of gluten to carry that label. "Wheat-free" does *not* necessarily mean "gluten-free," as ingredients like barley and rye are wheat-free but not gluten-free.

Source oats from a provider that can verify that their product is gluten-free. Crop and facility contamination can make a naturally gluten-free ingredient like oats contain gluten.

I call for coconut aminos as a "soy sauce" alternative because it's soy- *and* gluten-free. If soy isn't a concern for you but gluten is, try gluten-free tamari. If neither is a concern for you, *nama shoyu* or soy sauce will work great in any recipe that calls for coconut aminos.

Honey

All recipes in this book are vegan (as long as you use vegan ingredients) except ones that use honey (an animal product to vegans). I call for raw, unpastuerized honey to maintain nutritional benefits. Look for "wild-harvested" or "humanely harvested" if you want to know the treatment of the bees is gentle. Whenever honey is called for, you can substitute sticky sweeteners like maple syrup. Just know they'll alter flavor profiles.

For resources to help you make informed shopping choices, visit: **yumuniverse.com/pantry-to-plate-extras**

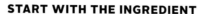

START WITH THE INGREDIENT

When you have celery in the crisper, tomatoes on the counter, or chard from the farmers' market and you aren't sure what to do with it, use the **Cook-by-Ingredient Index** on page 302 to inspire a plan of action.

SALT, SEASON & FLAVOR TO TASTE

The rule of thumb for salt, seasoning, and spices: Start with the lesser amount called for because you can always add more, not the other way around. Season and taste as you cook—train your taste buds.

Sea salt (delicious flavor plus beneficial trace minerals) and fresh-squeezed lemon juice round out and finish a recipe. Sea salt elevates flavor and aroma in both savory and sweet dishes. It tones down bitter notes and brightens sweetness. When we "salt to taste," we aren't really looking for salty flavor; we're looking to create depth and to make other flavors pop forward. Here's a test: Try a leaf of bitter radicchio plain and one sprinkled with a pinch of salt. The salted one will bring sweet notes forward and tone down bitterness. Sea salt can make a bland soup vibrant and a chocolate chip cookie sing. Note: Table salt is what yields unwanted "saltiness," so use sea salt. And salt savory dishes toward the end of cook time to allow other flavors to develop first. Unless otherwise specified, in this book, when I call for sea salt, I mean fine-ground.

Acids like lemon and vinegar create depth of flavor in meals as well. Try to use fresh lemon, lime, and orange juice versus the packaged stuff.

PLAN B

If you oversalt or overseason, or something doesn't come out right, instead of focusing on what didn't go as planned, think creatively. Sunken muffin? Make stuffing or bread pudding. Salty soup? Freeze half of it into flavor cubes to season future rice and grain dishes like Scrambles (page 36)—dilute the remaining soup with fresh, unsalted ingredients. And if you don't get to fresh ingredients before they start to perish, freeze them. Frozen fruits can always be used for smoothies, compotes, and baking, and most veggies can be used for making tasty veggie stocks and soups.

SERVING SIZES

Serving sizes vary in this book, but I usually begin with one to two people in mind—it's always easier to double or triple amounts called for to suit needs than it is to figure out what to do with loads of leftovers.

OILS

Some folks don't cook with oil and some do—these differences make the world go round, yes? I use oils in my cooking, but if you want to substitute, for savory meals, use veggie stock to sauté. For sweet baked treats, try bulky fruit substitutions like applesauce, avocado, and banana when oil is called for. When buying oils, look for "organic," "non-GMO," "cold-pressed," and "virgin" or "unrefined" for quality oils. And know that with every mention of coconut oil in this book, I mean cold-pressed, unrefined, virgin coconut oil, not refined.

THICKENING SAUCES & SOUPS

There are two ways I like to do this. One is using a starch/flour similar to cornstarch called arrowroot to make a slurry. Simply stir together 1½ teaspoons arrowroot starch/flour with ¼ cup (60 ml) water until dissolved and add it to warm sauces and soups (warmth activates thickening properties, while cooling finishes it). The other trick is the blend-and-bulk method. Take ¼ to 1 cup (60 to 240 ml) of the sauce, compote, or soup you are making, blend it until smooth, and add it back to your recipe to thicken.

APPLE CIDER VINEGAR IS YOUR BFF

Prolong the life of fresh berries so they're mold-free when you're ready to freestyle cook with them. When you bring them home, soak them in a mixing-bowl bath of cold water and 1 tablespoon apple cider vinegar for 5 to 7 minutes. Drain, quick rinse if you like (although I never really detect vinegar flavor if I don't), and store in the fridge. The acid in the vinegar inhibits mold growth and helps berries stay plump for weeks.

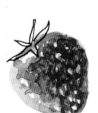

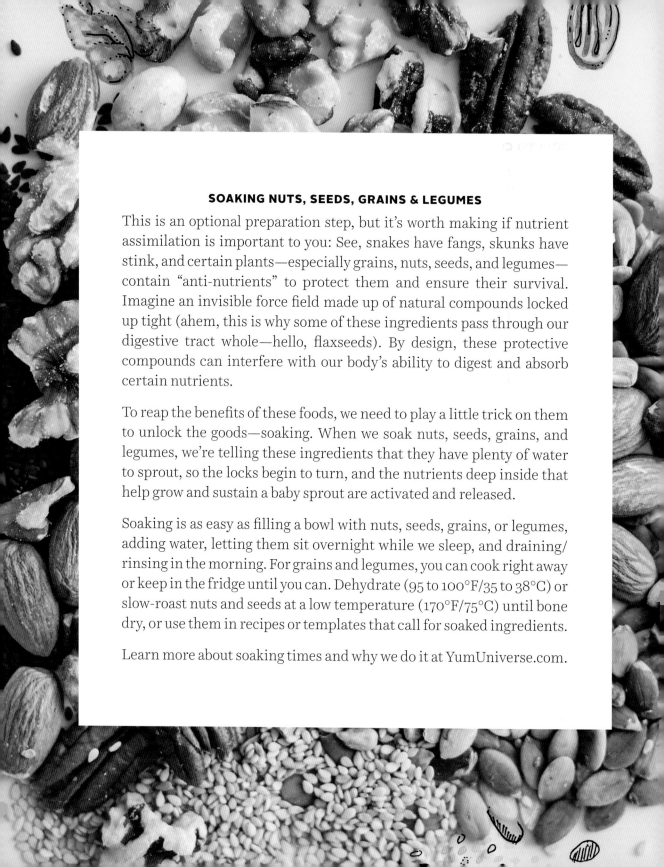

SOAKING NUTS, SEEDS, GRAINS & LEGUMES

This is an optional preparation step, but it's worth making if nutrient assimilation is important to you: See, snakes have fangs, skunks have stink, and certain plants—especially grains, nuts, seeds, and legumes—contain "anti-nutrients" to protect them and ensure their survival. Imagine an invisible force field made up of natural compounds locked up tight (ahem, this is why some of these ingredients pass through our digestive tract whole—hello, flaxseeds). By design, these protective compounds can interfere with our body's ability to digest and absorb certain nutrients.

To reap the benefits of these foods, we need to play a little trick on them to unlock the goods—soaking. When we soak nuts, seeds, grains, and legumes, we're telling these ingredients that they have plenty of water to sprout, so the locks begin to turn, and the nutrients deep inside that help grow and sustain a baby sprout are activated and released.

Soaking is as easy as filling a bowl with nuts, seeds, grains, or legumes, adding water, letting them sit overnight while we sleep, and draining/rinsing in the morning. For grains and legumes, you can cook right away or keep in the fridge until you can. Dehydrate (95 to 100°F/35 to 38°C) or slow-roast nuts and seeds at a low temperature (170°F/75°C) until bone dry, or use them in recipes or templates that call for soaked ingredients.

Learn more about soaking times and why we do it at YumUniverse.com.

Basic Cooking Techniques

HOW TO COOK GRAINS, LEGUMES & RICE

Preparing and cooking grains, legumes, beans, and rice from scratch is easier than you think. For legumes, beans, and grains, soak while you sleep—no need to soak rice. Rinse and cook, or store in the fridge until you can.

1. Soak grains, legumes, or beans in a bowl of water for 8 to 12 hours, then drain, rinse those soaked ingredients or unsoaked rice, and put in a pot with enough fresh water to cover by 1 inch (2.5 cm).

2. Bring to a boil, then reduce the heat to a simmer. Cover and let cook for the specified time or until the water or stock is absorbed.

3. Taste the cooked goods; if too firm, add a little more water and cook a little longer. If you taste again and the texture is perfect but there's still some water left, strain out the liquid and return to the pot.

4. Remove from the heat and allow to sit and finish, covered, for 5 to 10 minutes. Keep in mind that up to ¼ inch (6 mm) of water could absorb during rest time. For grains and rice, try not to peek, as trapped steam makes a fluffy texture.

5. Fluff with a fork and serve, or store in an airtight glass container in the fridge or freezer.

Isn't that easy? You can definitely use canned beans and legumes in a pinch, but try to make your own for maximum nutrition.

For extra trace minerals, place a 1-inch (2.5 cm) piece of kombu seaweed into the cooking water.

Beans

1 cup (200 g) beans
4 cups (960 ml) water or stock
Cook time: 45 to 90 minutes
Yields: 3+ cups (170+ g) cooked

Brown Rice

(Basmati, short, long grain)

1 cup (180 g) brown rice
3 cups (720 ml) water or stock
Cook time: 20 to 25 minutes
Yields: 2½ to 3 cups
(460 to 555 g) cooked

Buckwheat

1 cup (165 g) buckwheat
2 cups (480 ml) water or stock
Cook time: 10 to 15 minutes
Yields: 2 cups (340 g) cooked

Chickpeas

1 cup (200 g) chickpeas
4 cups (960 ml) water or stock
Cook time: 45 to 60 minutes
Yields: 3+ cups (495+ g) cooked

Lentils

(Red, green, brown,
French, beluga)

1 cup (190 g) lentils
2 cups (480 ml) water or stock
Cook time: 10 to 20 minutes
except red, which take 7 to
10 minutes
Yields: 3+ cups (600+ g) cooked

Quinoa

1 cup (170 g) quinoa
2½ cups (600 ml) water
or stock
Cook time: 10 to 15 minutes
Yields: 3 cups (555 g) cooked

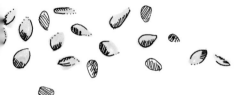

ROASTING & TOASTING

Roasting is done in the oven—a great technique for fruits, veggies, coconut, seeds, and nuts. *Toasting* is done in a dry skillet—perfect for nuts, seeds, grains, and treats like coconut flakes.

To roast: Preheat the oven to 350°F (180°C) and line a baking sheet with unbleached parchment paper or grease a glass, cast-iron, or ceramic roasting dish. Scatter the ingredients on the sheet (or in the pan) and make sure there is space around them to cook evenly. The smaller the chop, the shorter the cook time. Roast until easily pierced with a fork, but not mushy.

To toast: Scatter the ingredients in a dry skillet heated to medium-high, and stir until ingredients start to toast and smell fragrant, then remove from the heat.

STEAMING

You'll need a large pot with a steaming basket (or a footed sieve that fits inside the pot), and a lid. Fill the pot with water 1 inch (2.5 cm) below the bottom of the steaming basket and bring to a boil. Add your veggies to the basket and cover with the lid, but leave it a little bit open so steam can escape. For even cooking, it always helps to make sure the vegetables are chopped the same size. Steam until easily pierced with a fork, but not mushy.

DIFFERENT RANGES, DIFFERENT TEMPS

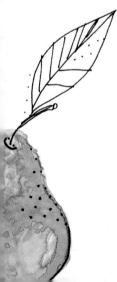

The templates and recipes in this book were developed on a gas range and tested on electric and gas ranges, because they're different animals. Note that instructions in this book favor a gas range. If you cook on an electric range, you can adjust (usually you'll go hotter) for stove-top cooking temperatures (for example: medium-high, low, etc.). Stick with oven temperature recommendations though (350°F/180°C, etc.)!

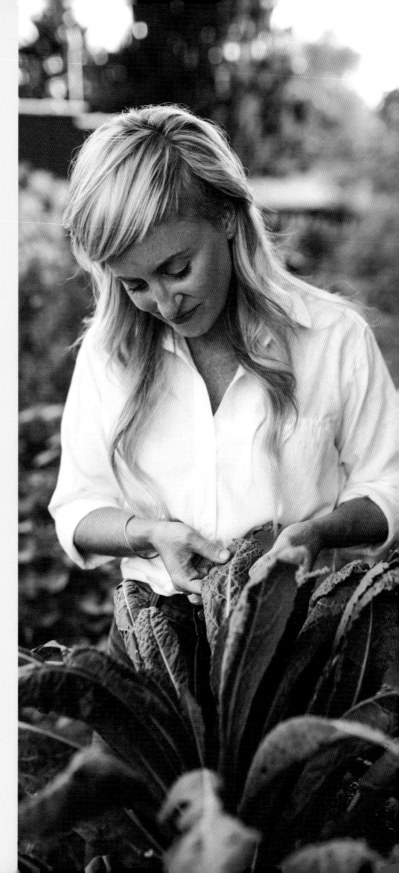

ROASTING & TOASTING TIMES

Coconut

3 to 5 minutes, and don't walk away—it can burn quickly

Nuts & Seeds

7 to 10 minutes

Grains

7 to 10 minutes

Fruit

30 to 45 minutes

Try firm fruits like pear and hearty berries like blueberry

Veggies

30 to 60 minutes

STEAMING TIMES

Peas, Broccoli & Cauliflower

3 to 7 minutes

You want vibrant color, easily pierced with a fork, but not mushy

Winter Squash & Root Veg

15 to 25 minutes

You want vibrant color, easily pierced with a fork, but not mushy

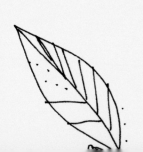

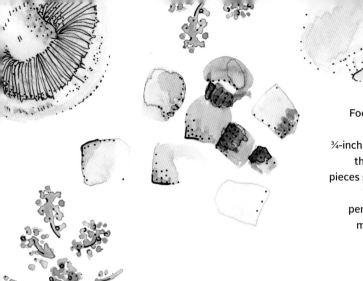

Chop

Foods cut into pieces with a knife or food processor. "Large chop" means that each piece is about a ¾-inch (2 cm) cube. A "medium chop" is about half that size; think dry kidney bean. Be sure to chop equal-sized pieces so food cooks evenly and in the same amount of time. The larger the chop, the longer it takes heat to penetrate and cook the goods—if you're in a hurry at mealtime, chop smaller pieces for faster cooking!

The Little Things

We all know that these are the things that make a significant difference—the way you simply prepare an ingredient can change the flavor and texture of a finished dish. Not *really* knowing the difference between a "chop" and a "dice" or how it affects a recipe can sometimes be enough to make someone abandon a home-cooked meal and pick up the phone for takeout instead. Here are some of the common terms you'll find in this book, some illustrations you can reference, and a little about why these common techniques are important for freestyle cooking.

Dice

Food cut into small cubes ¼ inch (6 mm) on all sides with a knife. Like chopping, dicing also helps add texture and ensures consistent, quick cooking for a dish.

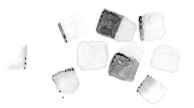

Grated/Shredded

Foods like carrots or ginger rubbed across a grating surface to make very fine, sometimes long-and-skinny pieces. A must to create maximum surface area for fermented vegetables, and the best way to incorporate raw, toothy root vegetables like beets into pancakes and muffins.

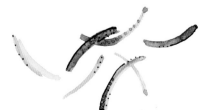

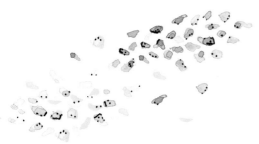

Mince

Fresh ingredients cut into very fine,
teeny-tiny pieces to evenly distribute and infuse
big color, texture, and flavor to a dish. When
mincing garlic, try sprinkling the clove with a
pinch of fine-ground sea salt to help prevent the
sugars from sticking to your knife.

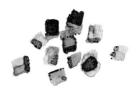

Zest

I love me some zest. It's the colored outer
portion of a citrus fruit peel—rich in fruit oils
and therefore flavor and fragrance.
Zest brightens dishes from cereal to cookies to
soups. To remove the zest, scrape a grater
or fruit zester across the peel. Or use a sharp
chef's knife to slice it off and mince into
tiny pieces. Avoid the white membrane (the pith)
beneath the peel—it's bitter.

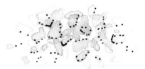

A Pinch

A small amount of a dry ingredient—
the amount that can be pinched between the
pointer finger and the thumb—roughly
$\frac{1}{8}$ to $\frac{1}{16}$ of a teaspoon. The goal is to train
the taste buds so you can rely more on a pinch
of this or that added to a recipe, tasting
as you go, than the recipe itself—freestyle!

Purée

Food processed or mashed until it's
as smooth as possible using a blender,
food processor, sieve, or masher.
Purées add moisture and natural sweetness
to baked goods, and they add
creamy flavor to cereals and soups.

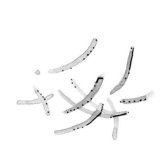

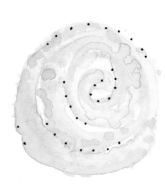

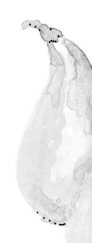

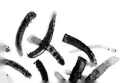

Tools & Ingredients

K eep your kitchen and pantry stocked so cooking is effortless and fun, but don't stress. While the items listed here are called for in many of the templates and recipes in this book, you don't need it all to freestyle cook. Shop for no-sugar-added and organic ingredients as much as possible. Use bulk bins for custom quantities and savings for herbs, spices, flours, grains, nuts, seeds, and more. Check out the resources on page 296 for shopping recs.

Basics

Baking sheet(s)

Wooden spoons

Silicone spatula(s)

Stainless steel

Pots & pans

Nonstick pan

Ceramic skillet

10- to 12-inch (25 to 30 cm) cast-iron skillet

Wood cutting board(s)

Paring knife

Chef's knife

Serrated knife

Plug-ins

Food processor

High-powered blender

Blender

Standing mixer

Prep

Measuring cups & spoons

Glass nesting bowls

Fine-mesh sieve (with feet)

Colander

Veggie peeler

Nice to Haves

Microplane zester

Mandoline

Dutch oven

Ice cream maker

Waffle iron

Tongs

Oils

Cold-pressed, unrefined coconut oil

Toasted sesame oil

Extra virgin olive oil

Grapeseed oil

Avocado oil

Vinegars

Apple cider vinegar, unpasteurized

Balsamic vinegar

Red wine vinegar

Rice vinegar

Sweeteners

Sucanat

Raw, unpasteurized honey

Maple syrup

Medjool dates

Gluten-Free Flours

Garbanzo bean flour

Brown rice flour

Sorghum flour

Almond flour

Oat flour

Dry Seasonings

Fine-ground sea salt

Black peppercorns

Ground cardamom

Cayenne pepper

Chili powder

Chipotle powder

Curry powder

Ground cinnamon

Ground coriander

Ground cumin

Red pepper flakes

Paprika

Ground nutmeg

Freezer

Tortillas

Berries & fruit

Veggies

Pantry & Fridge

Dijon and/or
whole-grain mustard

Marinated
artichoke hearts

Harissa chile pepper
paste (jar)

Sriracha hot sauce

Chickpea, adzuki bean,
or brown rice miso paste

Coconut aminos,
tamari, or soy sauce

Canned coconut milk

Gluten-free noodles
(soba, macaroni, etc.)

Tomato sauce

Veggie stock

Jam

Nutritional yeast

Coconut, flaked
or shredded

Plant Proteins

Brown rice

Buckwheat

Quinoa

Rolled oats

Millet

Lentils

Wild rice

Chickpeas

Beans (any kind)

Nuts & Seeds

Buy raw for all

Almonds

Hazelnuts

Hemp seeds

Pepitas

Cashews

Sunflower seeds

Sesame seeds

Pecans

Walnuts

Fresh Staples

Garlic

Onions or shallots

Bell peppers
(red, yellow, or orange)

Lemons & limes

Ginger

Fresh herbs

Apples or pears

Mushrooms

Dark, leafy greens

Lettuces

Squash, roots & tubers

Note: *Metric conversions
aren't always provided
in the templates, so please
see Measurements &
Conversions on page 298 for
metric info when needed.*

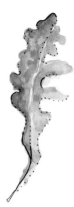

Freestyling
Flavors & Textures

Learning how to balance flavor and texture in a meal is important, but you don't have to go to cooking school to understand how it works.

There are five basic tastes used when cooking:

1 **Salty**: natural salt and sea veggies

2 **Sweet:** fruit, grains

3 **Sour:** fermented veg, sour fruits

4 **Bitter:** dark, leafy greens, herbs, spices

5 **Umami** ("pleasant savory flavor" in Japanese): earthy mushrooms, miso, grilled/seared/roasted foods

Ayurveda, which originated in India, is one of the world's oldest whole-body healing systems, and its approach to cooking includes:

Pungent: chile peppers, garlic

Astringent: raw fruits and veggies

Sometimes all five main tastes are employed, other times only one or two. But it's always about balance—flavors countering or harmonizing with each other to make a composed dish. A meal should be a layer cake of low notes (earthy, deep umami), middle notes (subtle, more fleeting flavors like those of raw veggies), and high notes (the brightness of fresh lemon or herbs), with a finish of roundness (the rug that pulls the entire living room together—a topping of cream or a simple pinch of salt). Thai food is a great example of flavor building in full effect: Think about a scrumptious curry where your taste buds get hit with sweet from coconut milk; salty and umami from soy sauce; spicy, bitter, earthy notes from herbs and chiles; and sour from a squeeze of lime. Yes.

We can start simply by choosing a few hero primary flavors and then choose secondary flavors that support and counter those primaries to balance the dish. For example, in the Italian-Style (Not)Meatballs on page 241, our primary ingredients are carrots (earthy and sweet), mushrooms (earthy and umami), and lentils (earthy and umami). They're already in harmony, so secondary and tertiary choices are onion and garlic (sour, pungent), sea salt (salty), herbs and black pepper (earthy and bitter), and smoked paprika (umami). You also want to think about texture as you flavor your dish. For the burger, you don't want uniform mush. Hearty, meaty texture comes from lentils; roasted carrots are soft and sticky; and the mushrooms have a chewy, sink-your-teeth-in bulk. They're delicious plain, but to really round out flavors, serve the final dish with a creamy lemon-based (acid and bright) dipping sauce from pages 186–187 (comforting) or with tomato sauce (sweet, acid).

The more you practice, the more creative, layered, and effortless your freestyle cooking will become. But if one of these notes ends up being too strong in a dish, try adding a contrasting flavor to even things out.

Salty: Add to enhance sweet flavors and balance bitterness. Think tomato jam, or the balance of bitter cabbage with salty brine for sauerkraut.

Sweet: Add to enhance salty flavors and balance sour, bitter, spicy, and umami notes in a dish. Think about the perfect salty-barely-sweet Asian noodle bowl, or salted caramel, and spicy hot chocolate.

Sour: Add to enhance salty and umami flavors, while balancing bitterness. Think about a squeeze of citrus over fresh-cooked lentils, or bitter endive with a yogurt-based dip.

Bitter: Add to enhance salty and umami notes in a meal. Think about seared bitter brussels sprouts tossed with a miso-mustard sauce.

Umami: Add to enhance sweetness and balance bitterness. Think about the deep, rich, complex flavor of Cashew-Almond Cheese Crumbles (page 133), or a creamy mushroom and kale soup.

Creating Rich Flavor
with Aromatics

S avory pantry-to-plate cooking begins with aromatics—the tasty foundation for flavorful dishes from all over the world. Aromatics are simply a combo of oil (or veggie stock), garlic, onions, ginger, celery, peppers, and/or carrots, and maybe some herbs and spices cooked at the kick start of a meal to impart incredible flavor and deep aroma to a completed dish. Once these starter ingredients begin heating up in a pot or skillet—"sweating" in chef speak—the kitchen fills with comforting smells, happy sounds, and a promise of tastiness ahead.

Without aromatics, a dish falls flat—they're essential for bringing depth of flavor. Try making a chana masala without garlic and ginger or a hearty stew without onions. Every bite will feel "hollow." Here are some simple, winning combos that'll build a solid foundation for any savory stove-top meal:

Chinese

Base: Oil + Scallions and/or Shallots + Garlic + Ginger

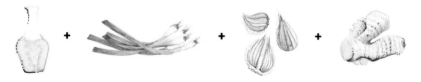

Supporting Cast: Chiles + Chives + Cilantro + Chinese Five-Spice + Star Anise

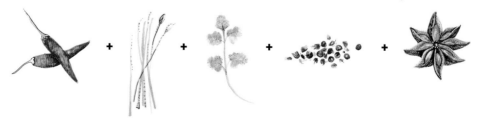

French (a.k.a. mirepoix)

Base: Oil + Onions + Carrots + Celery

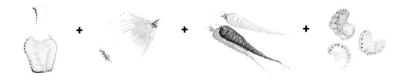

Supporting Cast: Parsley + Thyme + Bay Leaf + Herbes de Provence

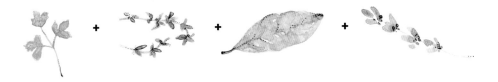

Indian

Base: Oil or Ghee + Onions + Garlic + Chiles + Ginger

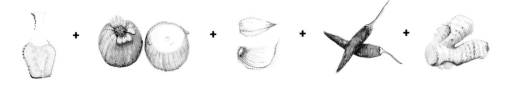

Supporting Cast: Tomatoes + Cardamom + Cumin + Curry (leaves, paste, ground) + Fenugreek + Cloves + Garam Masala + Turmeric

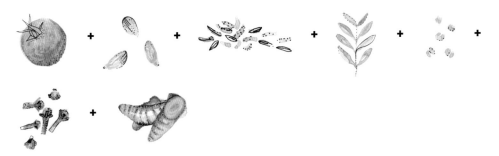

Italian (a.k.a. Soffrito)

Base: Oil + Onions + Carrots + Celery

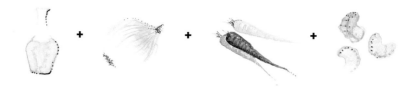

Supporting Cast: Garlic + Fennel + Bay Leaves + Parsley + Sage + Wine

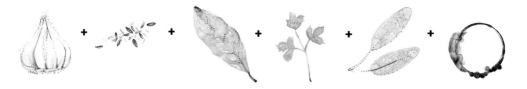

Latin (a.k.a. Sofrito)

Base: Oil + Onions + Garlic + Bell Peppers + Tomatoes

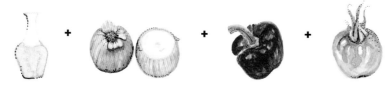

Supporting Cast: Chiles + Bay Leaves + Coriander + Cumin + Paprika + Cilantro + Wine + Vinegar

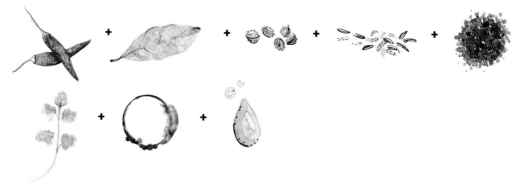

Middle Eastern

Base: Oil or Clarified Butter + Onions + Garlic + Tomatoes + Scallions + Raisins

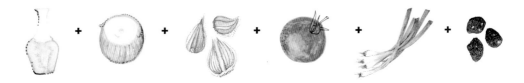

Supporting Cast: Ginger + Saffron + Turmeric + Cinnamon

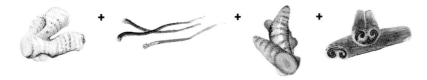

Thai

Base: Oil + Shallots + Garlic + Chiles

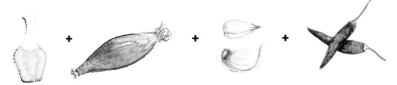

Supporting Cast: Galangal + Makrut Lime + Lemongrass + Coconut Milk

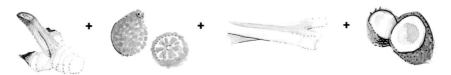

Herbs & Spices

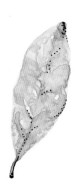

Are you one of those people who have an entire drawer of spices, but no idea how to use them? That used to be me. At some point out of curiosity, I started to sprinkle them on everything I made—veggies, grains, and beans. Why not? I realized that nothing ever got screwed up, everything ended up with enhanced flavor, and I was able to rock out dinner in 10 to 15 minutes. Soon, I was making my own spice blends and growing herbs in a windowsill garden.

No doubt about it, fresh herbs and spices are going to give you the best flavor, but premixed herb and seasoning blends are great for quick meal prep. Remember, they're supporting players used to enhance a dish, not dominate it. There are countless variations and no hard-and-fast rules, but with so many choices, you may not know where to begin.

WHAT PLAYS WELL TOGETHER?

The combinations listed here work well with all cooked grains, veg, legumes, beans, nuts, and seeds.

If you want to see how a mix will taste before you use it to cook a dish, finely chop and mix a tiny amount and stir into coconut oil, or a neutral-tasting dip or cheese. Or go for it, adding a little to your recipe at a time, seasoning to taste as you cook.

Many of the combos here, simply mixed with garlic and/or onion and/or fresh lemon, can transform a dish.

When buying premade herb and spice blends, look for organic, non-GMO products without unpronounceable, unrecognizable fillers or preservatives. You can dry your own herbs on a plate in the sun, so it's not unreasonable to expect store-bought to have the same simple ingredients, nothing extra.

Combos to Try

Allspice/red pepper flakes/black pepper/cinnamon/thyme

Anise/Szechuan peppercorn/cloves/fennel/coriander/cinnamon

Basil/thyme/oregano

Cinnamon/cardamom*

Chives/thyme/parsley/dill/tarragon/oregano/marjoram

Cinnamon/cocoa/cayenne*

Coriander/fennel

Cumin/coriander/chili powder/cinnamon/cilantro

Dill/chives/parsley

Marjoram/thyme/oregano

Mint/basil*

Nutmeg/coriander/cinnamon/cloves/cumin/cardamom/paprika

Paprika/cumin/chipotle/mustard

Parsley/basil/chives

Sage/thyme/rosemary

Sumac/thyme/sesame seeds

Tarragon/parsley

Thyme/savory/marjoram/rosemary/lavender

Turmeric/coriander/cumin/fenugreek/red pepper flakes

Try in sweet and savory dishes

Premixed Blends

Stock a few of these in your pantry for easy, quick meals:

Chinese five-spice

Curry powder

Garam masala

Italian seasoning

Herbes de Provence

Jerk seasoning

Montreal steak seasoning

Taco seasoning

Za'atar spice blend

A Little Goes a Long Way

Some herbs and spices pack a lot of flavor and should be used sparingly. Always start with a pinch, and add more to taste with the following:

Allspice

Anise

Cardamom

Cayenne pepper

Chipotle powder

Cloves

Nutmeg

Red pepper flakes

Rosemary

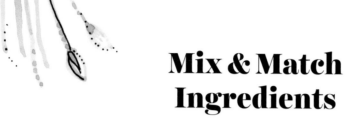

Mix & Match Ingredients

Pantry-to-plate cooking is all about creating a dish using interchangeable ingredients—cooking intuitively and confidently without a recipe. To keep it easy, in some templates I may call for a general group of ingredients like "Hearty Greens" or "Citrus." Use the lists here to familiarize yourself with what each group includes.

Alliums

Chive

Garlic

Leek

Onion

Ramp

Scallion

Shallot

Berries

Blackberry

Blueberry

Raspberry

Strawberry

Wineberry

Brassicas

Broccoli

Brussels sprouts

Cabbage

Citrus (sour)

Grapefruit

Lemon

Lime

Citrus (sweet)

Orange

Clementine

Kumquat

Tangerine

Pome Fruit

Apple

Pear

Quince

Hearty Greens

Mustard greens

Collard greens

Kale

Chard

Beet greens

Turnip greens

Grains & Pseudograins

Buckwheat

Millet

Oat

Quinoa

Rice

Sorghum

Tender Greens

Arugula

Watercress

Spinach

Chicories

Belgian endive

Escarole

Frisée

Radicchio

Dandelion

Lettuces

Butterhead

Romaine

Red leaf

Green leaf

Mixed greens

Mushrooms

Cremini

Oyster

Portobello

Maitake

Shiitake

White button

Pulses

Adzuki beans

Black beans

Black-eyed peas

Cannellini beans

Chickpeas

Kidney beans

Lentils

Mung beans

Pinto beans

Split peas

Roots & Tubers

Beet

Carrot

Jicama

Parsnip

Purple potato

Radish

Rutabaga

Sweet potato

Turnip

Yam

Stone Fruit

Apricot

Cherry

Peach

Plum

Nectarine

Summer Melon

Cantaloupe

Honeydew

Watermelon

Summer Squash

Cousa squash

Eight-ball zucchini

Green zucchini

Patty pan

Tatuma squash

Yellow squash

Yellow zucchini

Zephyr squash

Winter Squash

Acorn

Buttercup

Butternut

Carnival

Delicata

Hubbard

Kabocha

Pumpkin

Red kuri

Sweet dumpling

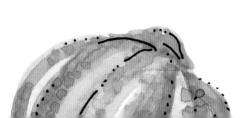

Homemade Staples:
Sauces & Dressings

Skip the preservatives and sugar from store-bought sauces and dressings—make your own. Sure, packaged goods make for quick and easy cooking, but nothing beats homemade. Store in the fridge for seven to ten days, and if the sauce separates, shake it before serving. Freeze in batches or in flavor cubes (use an ice cube tray) for a few months—thaw and shake or reheat to enjoy.

Savory Marinade

Umami flavor for veggies, rice, grains, and more

¼ cup (60 ml) coconut aminos (or soy sauce or tamari)

2 tablespoons extra virgin olive oil

2 tablespoon ume plum vinegar

1 teaspoon miso

¼ teaspoon liquid smoke

Sea salt to taste

Fresh-cracked black pepper to taste

Whisk all ingredients together—blend for a creamy version.

Makes ½ cup (120 ml)

Butternut Squash Sauce

Try on macaroni noodles (from page 186 template)

2 cups (410 g) peeled, seeded, diced, and steamed/roasted butternut squash

½ cup (70 g) cashews, soaked 4 to 6 hours, drained, and rinsed

½ cup (120 ml) water

2 teaspoons nutritional yeast

2 teaspoons unrefined coconut oil (optional)

1 teaspoon fresh lemon juice

½ teaspoon sea salt, or more to taste

Blend all ingredients together until smooth.

Makes 2+ cups (480+ ml)

Chipotle Cream

Prepare for addiction (from page 186 template)

2½ cups (350 g) cashews, soaked 4 to 6 hours, drained, and rinsed

½ cup (120 ml) water

2 teaspoons fresh lime juice

¼ teaspoon grated lime zest

2 tablespoons packed fresh cilantro leaves

¼ teaspoon chipotle powder

½ to 1 teaspoon sea salt, to taste

Blend all ingredients together until smooth.

Makes 3+ cups (720+ ml)

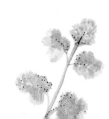

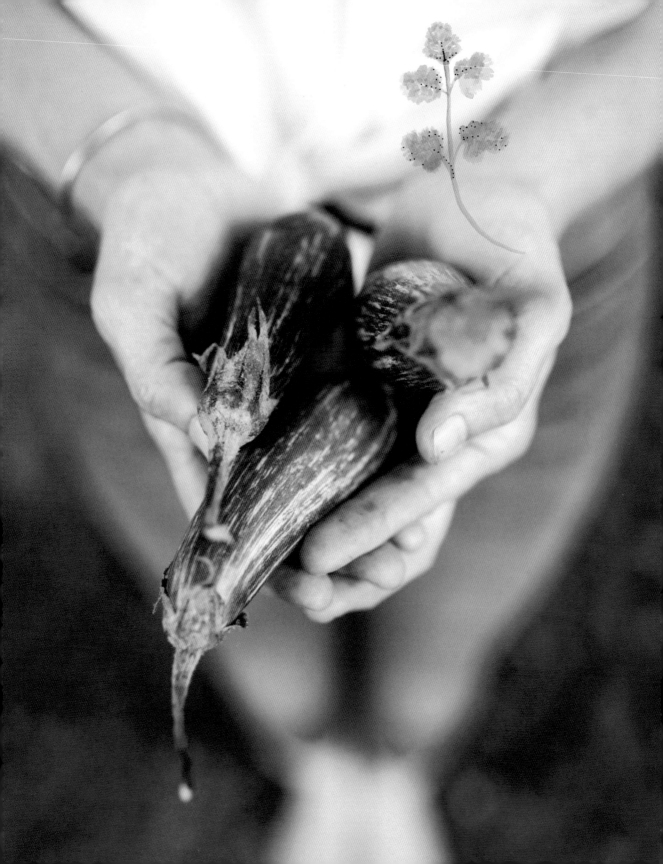

Orange-Sesame Sauce

Asian-style dip/sauce for rice, grains, or veg

¼ cup (60 ml) coconut aminos (or soy sauce or tamari)

3 tablespoons chopped scallions

2 to 3 tablespoons maple syrup, to taste

1 tablespoon cashew or almond butter

1 tablespoon fresh orange juice

1 tablespoon rice vinegar

1 tablespoon toasted sesame oil

1 garlic clove, minced

1 teaspoon grated orange zest

1 teaspoon toasted sesame seeds (optional)

¼ teaspoon peeled, grated fresh ginger

¼ teaspoon red pepper flakes

Sea salt to taste

Whisk all ingredients together—blend for a creamy version.

Makes 1+ cup (240+ ml)

Chimichurri

A refreshing dip/sauce for rice, grains, or roasted veg

½ cup (30 g) chopped fresh parsley leaves

½ cup (120 ml) extra virgin olive oil

2 tablespoons apple cider or red wine vinegar

3 garlic cloves, minced

1 tablespoon chopped fresh oregano

1 tablespoon minced red onion or shallot

2 teaspoons fresh lemon or lime juice

½ teaspoon grated lemon or lime zest

½ teaspoon red pepper flakes

½ teaspoon sea salt, or more to taste

Whisk or pulse all ingredients together in the food processor—blend for a creamy version.

Makes ¾ to 1 cup (180 to 240 ml)

Smoky BBQ Sauce

Smoke-pit flavor for rice, grains, veg, and more

1 cup (50 g) sun-dried tomatoes, soaked 1 to 2 hours and drained

1 cup (240 ml) water

¼ cup (60 ml) apple cider vinegar

¼ cup (50 g) Sucanat

1 large garlic clove, sautéed for 3 minutes

2 to 3 tablespoons raw, unpasteurized honey (or Sucanat), to taste

2 heaping tablespoons diced white onion, sautéed for 5 to 7 minutes

2 tablespoons fresh lemon juice

1 tablespoon coconut aminos (or soy sauce or tamari)

½ to 1 teaspoon liquid smoke or 1 teaspoon smoked paprika (optional), to taste

½ to 1 teaspoon sea salt, to taste

Fresh-cracked black pepper to taste

Two pinches cayenne pepper (optional)

Blend all ingredients together until smooth.

Makes 3+ cups (720+ ml)

Enchilada Sauce

Zesty dip or sauce for rice, grains, and veg

3 tablespoons unrefined coconut oil

½ yellow onion, diced

2 large tomatoes, blanched (optional) and chopped

1½ cups (360 ml) low-sodium vegetable stock

3 garlic cloves, minced

3 tablespoons chili powder

2 tablespoons gluten-free all-purpose flour

1 tablespoon fresh lime juice

2 teaspoons cacao/cocoa powder

1½ teaspoons sea salt

1 teaspoon ground cumin

¼ teaspoon ground coriander

In a skillet heated to medium-high, add the oil and sauté the onion for 5 minutes. Add the tomatoes and cook down for 10 minutes. Add the remaining ingredients, bring to a boil, reduce the heat, and simmer for 10 minutes. Blend and serve.

Makes 2+ cups (480+ ml)

Vinaigrette

Dress a salad, marinate roasted veg, and toss with grains or rice

¾ cup (120 ml) extra virgin olive oil

¼ cup (60 ml) wine vinegar (any kind)

1 large shallot (optional), minced

Sea salt and fresh-cracked black pepper to taste

Whisk all ingredients together or blend until smooth.

Makes 1 cup (240 ml)

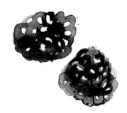

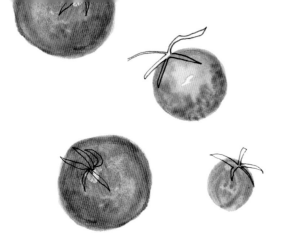

Cauliflower Cream

Cheese-like comfort sauce (from page 186 template)

2 cups (215 g) cauliflower florets, steamed or roasted

½ cup (70 g) cashews or sunflower seeds, soaked 4 to 6 hours, drained, and rinsed

½ cup (120 ml) water

2 garlic cloves, roasted

2 teaspoons nutritional yeast (optional)

2 teaspoons unrefined coconut oil (optional)

1 teaspoon fresh lemon juice

½ teaspoon sea salt, or more to taste

Fresh-cracked black pepper to taste

Blend all ingredients together until smooth.

Makes 2+ cups (480+ ml)

Cashew Cream

The dairy-free holy grail (from page 186 template)

2½ cups (350 g) cashews, soaked 4 to 6 hours, drained, and rinsed

¾ cup (180 ml) water, plus more if needed

2 teaspoons fresh lemon juice

1 teaspoon sea salt, or more to taste

Blend all ingredients together until smooth and, if needed, add more water ¼ cup (60 ml) at a time to reach the consistency you want.

Makes 3+ cups (720+ ml)

Maudie's Tomato Sauce

Inspired by my grandma's legendary tomato sauce (sans meat)

2 tablespoons unrefined coconut oil

1 large yellow onion, diced

3 to 4 garlic cloves, minced

8 large tomatoes, blanched (optional), peeled, and chopped

½ cup (120 ml) dry red wine (optional)

2 tablespoons packed fresh basil

½ teaspoon liquid smoke (optional)

2 teaspoons sea salt, plus more to taste

Fresh-cracked black pepper to taste

In a large pot heated to medium-high, add the oil and sauté the onion for 7 minutes, then add the garlic and stir for 3 more minutes. Add the tomatoes, wine (if using), basil, and liquid smoke (if using) and bring to a boil. Reduce the heat, cover, and simmer for 30 minutes. Add the salt and pepper and enjoy.

Makes 3+ cups (720+ ml)

Butterscotch

Takes sweet treats and fruit to the next level

1 tablespoon arrowroot starch/flour

¼ cup (60 ml) water

1½ cups (360 ml) canned coconut milk

1 cup (190 g) Sucanat

½ cup (120 ml) brown rice syrup

3 tablespoons unrefined coconut oil

½ teaspoon sea salt

½ teaspoon vanilla extract

In a cup, stir together the arrowroot and water until thoroughly dissolved and set aside. In a large saucepan heated to medium-high, whisk together all remaining ingredients except the arrowroot slurry. Once the mixture boils, whisk in the arrowroot slurry. Remove from the heat but continue to whisk vigorously for 1 minute. As it cools, the butterscotch will thicken. Serve warm.

Makes 3+ cups (720+ ml)

Supergreen Pesto

Herby cheese-like flavor for rice, grains, veg, toast

1 cup (15 g) lightly packed kale

1 cup (40 g) packed fresh basil

½ cup (120 ml) extra virgin olive oil

¼ cup (35 g) pine nuts, toasted

2 garlic cloves

1 tablespoon nutritional yeast

2 teaspoons fresh lemon juice

½ teaspoon sea salt

Fresh-cracked black pepper to taste (optional)

Pulse all ingredients in a food processor until mixed, but not blended. Serve or chill.

Makes 1 to 2 cups (240 to 480 ml)

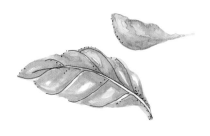

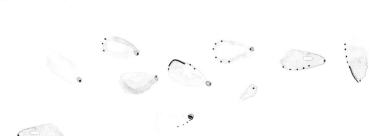

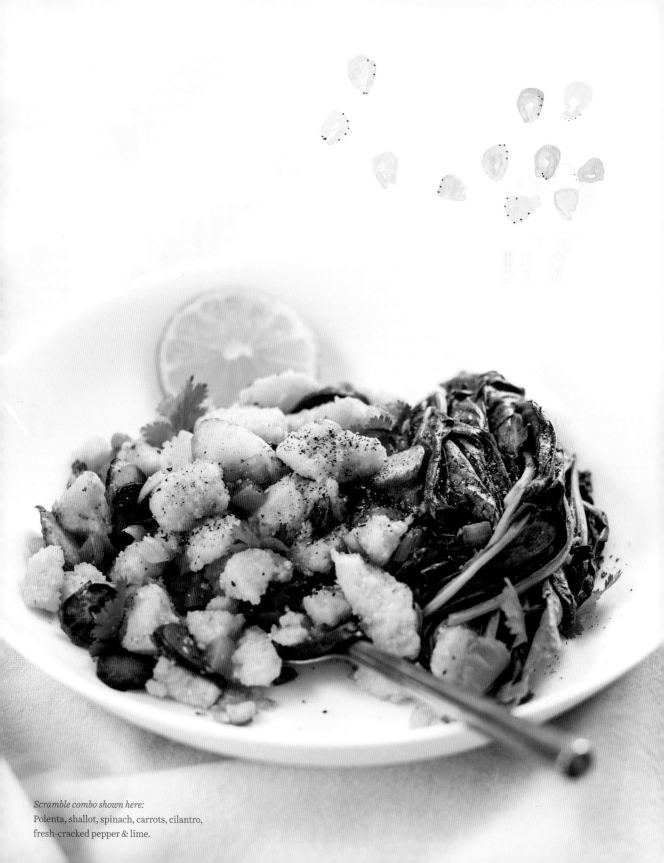

Scramble combo shown here:
Polenta, shallot, spinach, carrots, cilantro,
fresh-cracked pepper & lime.

Good Morning, YumUniverse!

WHEN I HAD TO MAKE CHANGES IN MY DIET, one of my first questions was "What on earth will I eat for breakfast?!"

This was quickly followed by a sharp pang of FOMO (fear of missing out) for what I thought was the end of Sunday brunch. But instead of indulging in complaining, I got creative and found that breakfast and brunch could offer more than I ever imagined as soon as I started adding more of the good stuff to the routine. Pancakes are a canvas for myriad flavors, there are countless breakfast scramble combinations, and you can even make a variety of flavorful milks and probiotic-rich yogurts without a single cow!

Use the following pages as a springboard—if animal products like eggs and milk are part of your life, by all means, add them to these recipes and templates.

Scrambles

1 TO 2 SERVINGS
COOK TIME: 15 TO 35 MINUTES

A Scramble is the perfect last-minute, I-don't-want-to-think-too-hard-about-it, one-pot meal.

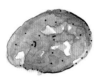

What you need no matter what:

1 tablespoon unrefined coconut oil, grapeseed oil, or avocado oil

1 to 3 garlic cloves, minced (optional)

½ teaspoon fine-ground sea salt, plus more to taste

1 In a skillet heated to medium, add the **oil** and sauté Dense Veg (if using) for 10 to 20 minutes, until easily pierced with a fork, but still firm.

Dense Veg

½ TO 1 CUP CHOPPED TOTAL
Choose one or combine, or skip altogether

Sweet potatoes	Beets
Winter squash	Potatoes

2 Now, add Veggies and sauté over medium heat for 3 to 5 minutes, until softened and vibrant in color. Then fold in Texture and sauté for 1 minute.

Veggies ---- *and* ---> Texture

1 TO 2 CUPS CHOPPED TOTAL
Choose two or more

Onion (any kind)	Cauliflower
Shallot	Eggplant
Bell pepper (any kind)	Green peas (no need to chop!)
Celery	Mushrooms
Asparagus	Summer squash
Broccoli	Tomatoes
	Carrots

¼ TO 1½ CUPS TOTAL
Choose one or combine—see how to cook beans, legumes, and grains on page 11

Oats, uncooked

Precook the following ingredients:

Beans (any kind)

Buckwheat, hulled

Chickpeas

Lentils

Millet

Polenta

Quinoa

Rice (any kind)

3   Fold Green Stuff (if using) into the Scramble. Add the **garlic** if you like; sauté for 3 minutes.

Green Stuff

Choose one or combine, or skip altogether

1 to 4 tablespoons chopped fresh herbs (any kind)

1 to 2 cups (15 to 60 g) chopped dark, leafy greens

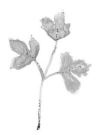

4   Choose either one Sauce or one Seasoning (if using)—we want to let just one be the hero. Fold into your scramble. Sauté for 1 to 2 minutes.

Sauce ----- *or* -----→ Seasoning

¼ TO ½ CUP (60 TO 120 ML) TOTAL
Choose one or skip altogether

2 TEASPOONS TO 2 TABLESPOONS, TO TASTE
Choose one or skip altogether

Smoky BBQ Sauce (page 30)	Coconut aminos (or tamari or soy sauce)	BBQ dry rub	Montreal steak seasoning
Chipotle Cream (page 28)	Savory Marinade (page 28)	Ethiopian berbere spice	Old Bay seasoning
Cashew Cream (page 32)	Enchilada Sauce (page 31)	Cajun mix	Taco/fajita seasoning mix
Cauliflower Cream (page 32)	Salsa	Curry powder	Za'atar spice blend
	Supergreen Pesto (page 33)	Garam masala	
		Jamaican jerk seasoning	

5   Add the **salt** or more to taste and any Finishing Touches (if using; you choose the amount).

Finishing Touches

Choose one or combine, or skip altogether

Fresh-cracked black pepper	Coconut cream	Fresh lemon juice	Toasted nuts or seeds (any kind)
Cashew Cream (page 32)	Scallions	Cashew-Almond Cheese Crumbles (page 133)	Avocado
	Fresh herbs, chopped		

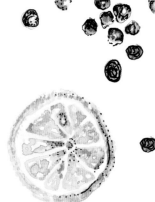

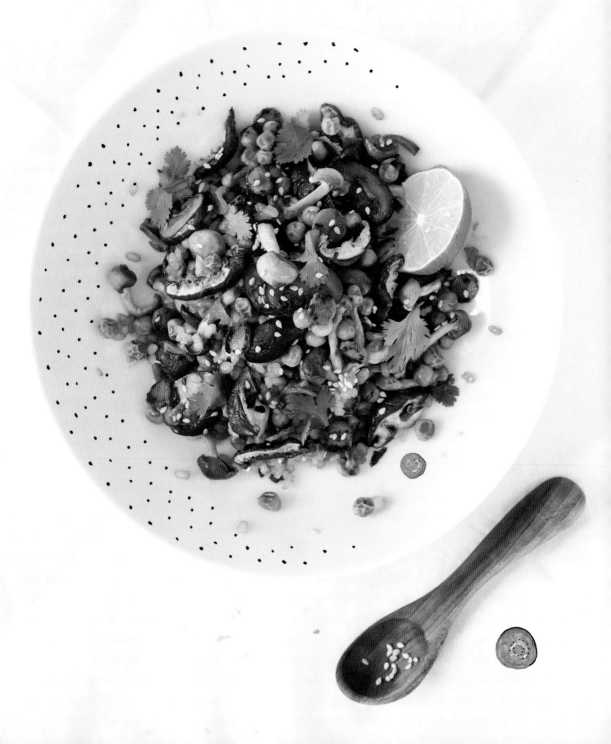

Many-Mushroom Scramble *with* Orange-Sesame Sauce

Vibrant Orange-Sesame Sauce and a variety of mushrooms make this easy stir-fry scramble an instant favorite.

SERVES 1 TO 2

1 tablespoon unrefined coconut oil

1 cup (70 g) assorted mushrooms (portobello, baby bella, shiitake, maitake, crimini, etc.), sliced

½ cup (70 g) green peas

¼ cup (40 g) diced shallots

¼ cup (30 g) sliced carrots

1 cup (195 g) cooked brown rice (½ cup/95 g dry; see page 11 for tips)

1 to 2 garlic cloves, minced

Small handful fresh cilantro, plus more for garnish

¼ cup (60 ml) Orange-Sesame Sauce (page 30) or any Asian-style stir-fry sauce you like

½ teaspoon sea salt, plus more to taste

½ cup (70 g) raw, unsalted cashews, toasted

1 lime

1 tablespoon sesame seeds, toasted

1. In a skillet heated to medium, add the coconut oil and sauté the mushrooms, peas, shallots, and carrots for 3 to 5 minutes, until softened and vibrant in color.

2. Then fold in the rice and sauté for 1 minute. Add the garlic and cilantro and sauté for 3 minutes.

3. Fold the Orange-Sesame Sauce into your scramble and sauté for 1 to 2 minutes. Add the salt, fold in the cashews, and top with a little more cilantro, a squeeze of fresh lime juice, and sesame seeds. Serve warm.

Pesto Chickpea & Quinoa Scramble

I make this scramble at least once a week with whatever grains
or legumes I have cooked in the fridge and the veggies
I have lying around—it's all about the Supergreen Pesto here
(which keeps for a while in the fridge—hint, hint).

SERVES 1 TO 2

1 tablespoon unrefined
coconut oil

1 cup (70 g) broccoli florets

½ cup (80 g) diced white onion

½ cup (85 g) cooked chickpeas
(roughly ¼ cup/50 g dry;
see page 11 for tips)

½ cup (90 g) cooked quinoa
(roughly ¼ cup/40 g dry;
see page 11 for tips)

½ cup (8 g) packed lacinato kale,
stems removed, chopped
or chiffonade

¼ to ½ cup (60 to 120 ml)
Supergreen Pesto (page 33)
to taste

½ teaspoon sea salt,
or more to taste

Fresh lemon juice (optional)

Avocado, sliced or diced

Handful fresh basil

1 In a skillet heated to medium, add the coconut oil and sauté the broccoli
   and onion for 3 to 5 minutes, until softened and vibrant in color. Then fold
   in the chickpeas and quinoa and sauté for 1 minute. Add the kale and sauté
   for 3 minutes.

2 Fold the Supergreen Pesto into your scramble and sauté for 1 to 2 minutes.

3 Add the salt. Remove from the heat, top with a squeeze of lemon juice
   (if using) and the avocado and basil, and serve warm.

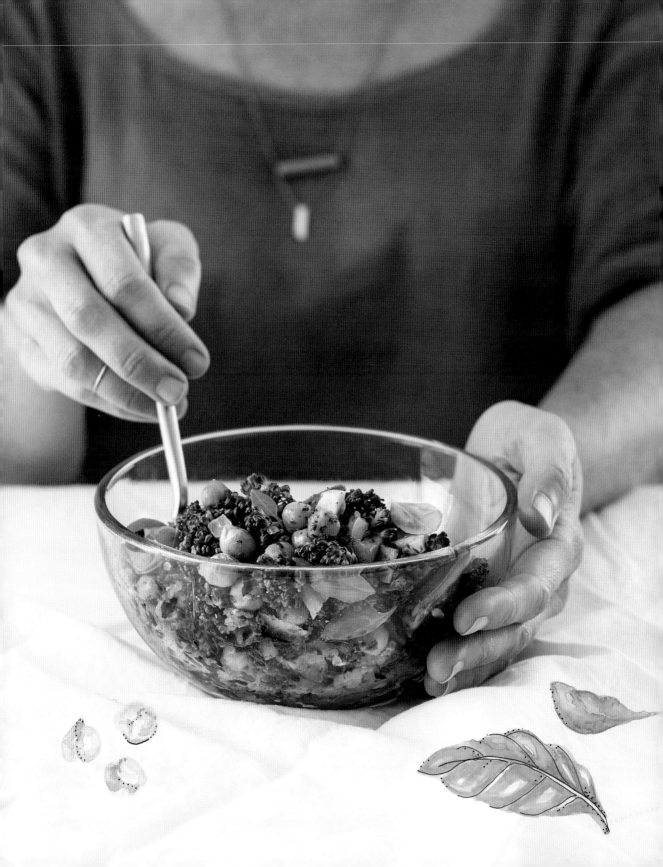

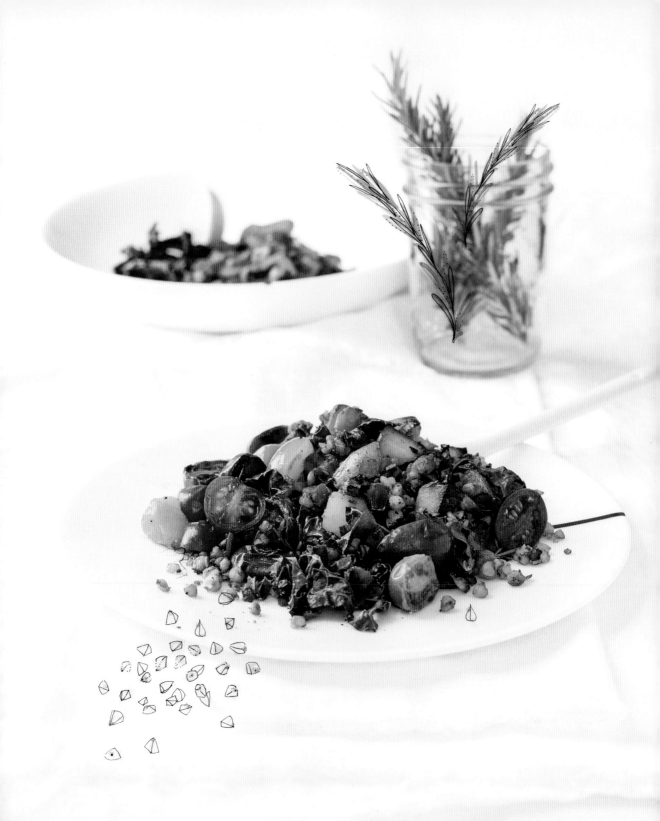

Herbed Potato, Kale & Buckwheat Scramble

I'm always adding colorful veggies to classic basics like a hash browns recipe. This scramble takes roasted potatoes from side dish to main course in minutes.

SERVES 1 TO 2

1 tablespoon unrefined coconut oil

1 cup (150 g) diced or shredded red-skinned and/or purple potatoes

½ cup (75 g) diced red bell pepper

½ cup (80 g) diced yellow onion

½ cup (75 g) halved cherry tomatoes

¾ cup (125 g) cooked hulled buckwheat groats (roughly ½ cup/80 g dry; see page 11)

½ cup (15 g) packed lacinato kale, stems removed, chopped or chiffonade

1 tablespoon fresh rosemary, chopped or whole leaf

½ teaspoon sea salt, or more to taste

Fresh-cracked black pepper

Fresh lemon juice

1. In a skillet heated to medium, add the coconut oil and sauté the potatoes for 20 minutes, until easily pierced with a fork but firm, not mushy.

2. Add the red pepper, onion, and tomatoes and sauté over medium heat for 3 to 5 minutes, until softened and vibrant in color.

3. Fold in the buckwheat and sauté for 1 minute, then fold the kale and rosemary into the scramble and sauté for 3 minutes. Add the salt, generous fresh-cracked pepper, and a squeeze of fresh lemon juice. Serve warm.

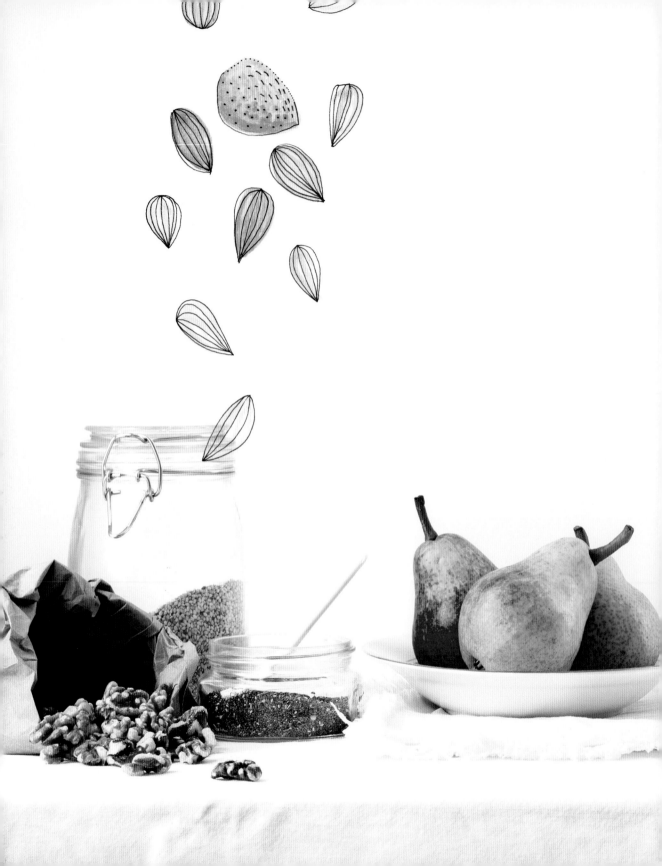

Granola

Granola is great for quick breakfasts, on-the-go snacking, and adding texture to Nice Creams (page 279) and Yogurts (page 94), and it even makes a thoughtful gift.

Try fennel and orange for a unique twist. Keep it classic with cinnamon and cranberries, or go artisanal with ground tea or Brazil nuts. Grain-free? Use almond flour. Nut-free? Try quinoa or brown rice flakes (they look like rolled oats). Olive oil lends rich, toasty, savory notes that play well with sweet elements. Try a splash of aged balsamic vinegar in a chocolate version, probably with white chocolate chips and cherries—infinite possibilities.

Just be sure to check out page 101 for homemade Dairy-Free Milks you can serve with your granola, too.

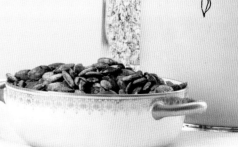
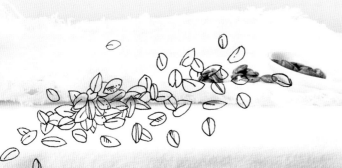

Granola

6+ SERVINGS
COOK TIME: 20 TO 40 MINUTES

Granola is *so* pantry-to-plate cooking because countless tasty combinations are possible, and it's super easy to make.

What you need no matter what:

½ to 1 teaspoon sea salt

1 Preheat the oven to 300°F (150°C). In a large bowl, combine Crunch, Nuts & Seeds (if using), Sweet, and Oil (if using).

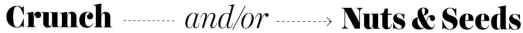

Crunch ----- *and/or* -----> ## Nuts & Seeds

3 CUPS TOTAL
Choose one or combine

Blanched almond flour (grain-free)

Hazelnut flour/meal (grain-free)

Brown rice flakes

Oats (old-fashioned rolled or steel cut)

Hulled buckwheat groats

Quinoa flakes

1½ CUPS TOTAL
Choose one or combine, or skip altogether; raw and unsalted

Almonds

Sesame seeds (best in small amounts)

Brazil nuts

Hazelnuts

Sunflower seeds

Pepitas

Walnuts

Poppy seeds (best in small amounts)

Sweet ----- *and/or* -----> ## Oil

¾ TO 1 CUP (180 TO 240 ML) TOTAL
Choose one or combine

Blackstrap molasses

Raw, unpasteurized honey

Brown rice syrup

Maple syrup

¼ CUP (60 ML) TOTAL
Optional

Unrefined coconut oil

Grapeseed oil

Extra virgin olive oil

Sunflower seed oil

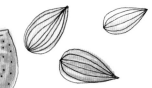

2 Add Flavors and the **salt** to taste and stir. Spread mixture in an even layer about ¼ inch (6 mm) thick onto a rimmed baking sheet. Give it a light press for chunky granola.

Flavors Optional

Choose any of these in combination **OR** ----------------------> *Choose one of these by itself*

2 to 4 tablespoons cacao nibs

¼ teaspoon ground cardamom

¼ teaspoon cayenne pepper

1 to 2 teaspoons ground cinnamon

¼ teaspoon ground cloves

¼ teaspoon fresh-ground nutmeg

1 teaspoon extract (almond, chocolate, hazelnut, vanilla)

1 to 3 tablespoons grated citrus zest

3 tablespoons unsalted nut or seed butter

2 to 3 tablespoons cocoa/cacao powder

2 tablespoons ground coffee

1 teaspoon balsamic vinegar

1 teaspoon orange blossom or rosewater

1 teaspoon fennel seed

½ to 1 teaspoon ground ginger (or 1 to 2 teaspoons peeled, minced fresh ginger)

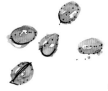

3 Bake for 15 to 20 minutes and then stir (if not using oil, bake for 10 minutes). If using Special Additions, add them to the granola and stir. Press again and bake for 15 to 20 more minutes (if not using oil, bake for 10 more minutes). Granola will harden as it cools.

Special Additions Choose as many as you like, or skip altogether

¼ to 1 cup (35 to 140 g) raw, unsalted cashews

2 tablespoons chia seeds

½ to 1 cup (40 to 80 g) dried coconut (shredded or flakes)

1 to 2 tablespoons tea leaves, ground in coffee/spice grinder (chai, Earl Grey, etc.)

¼ to 1 cup (25 to 100 g) pecans

¼ to ½ cup (35 to 70 g) raw, unsalted pine nuts

½ teaspoon fresh rosemary

1 to 2 teaspoons fresh thyme

4 Once cooled, transfer to a large bowl, break apart, and add any Finishing Touches, if you like. Make sure the granola is cool if adding chocolate or it will melt into the mix. Impatient? Pop the granola in the freezer to expedite cooling. Store in an airtight container in the pantry or fridge for 4 to 8 weeks.

Finishing Touches Choose as many as you like, or skip altogether

1 to 2 cups dried fruit (pome, berries, tropical)

1 cup (135 g) raw macadamia nuts, chopped

½ cup (15 g) crispy brown rice cereal

½ cup (90 g) chopped chocolate or chocolate chips (dark or white)

½ cup (80 g) crystallized ginger, chopped

½ cup (80 g) heat-sensitive seeds (hemp, flax)

½ cup (10 g) popped/puffed grains (amaranth, brown rice, millet, quinoa)

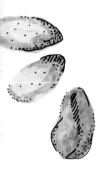

Dark Chocolate, Cherry & Brazil Nut Granola

Earthy, chocolaty cacao; red-wine-tasting cacao nibs; tart, sweet, chewy cherries; and creamy crunch from Brazil nuts taste like eating-out decadence, yet this recipe can be whipped up in the comfort of your own kitchen in no time. Serve with Coconut Yogurt (page 94) and cherry Compote (page 90), homemade Dairy-Free Milk (page 101), or some Nice Cream (page 279).

SERVES 8+

3 cups (240 g) rolled oats

1 cup (240 ml) maple syrup

1 cup (135 g) raw, unsalted Brazil nuts, chopped

½ cup (50 g) raw, unsalted walnuts, chopped

¼ cup (35 g) cacao nibs

¼ cup (60 ml) unrefined coconut oil

3 tablespoons cocoa/cacao powder

1½ teaspoons ground cinnamon

1 teaspoon chocolate extract (optional)

1 teaspoon vanilla extract

¾ teaspoon sea salt

¼ teaspoon cayenne pepper (optional)

1 cup (85 g) flaked coconut

2 tablespoons chia seeds

1 cup (160 g) dried cherries (cook's choice: sweetened or unsweetened)

½ cup (15 g) crispy brown rice cereal

1. Preheat the oven to 300°F (150°C). In a large bowl, combine the oats, maple syrup, Brazil nuts, walnuts, cacao nibs, coconut oil, cacao powder, cinnamon, extracts, salt, and cayenne.

2. Spread the mixture on a rimmed baking sheet in an even layer about ¼ inch (6 mm) thick. Give it a light press and bake for 20 minutes.

3. At the 20-minute mark, stir the coconut flakes and chia seeds into your granola until thoroughly incorporated. Lightly press down again and bake for 15 to 20 more minutes, until golden brown and well toasted. The granola continues baking when you pull it from the oven, and it hardens on the baking sheet as it cools.

4. Once cooled, transfer to a large bowl, break apart, and add the cherries and crispy brown rice cereal. Store in an airtight container in the pantry or fridge for 4 to 8 weeks.

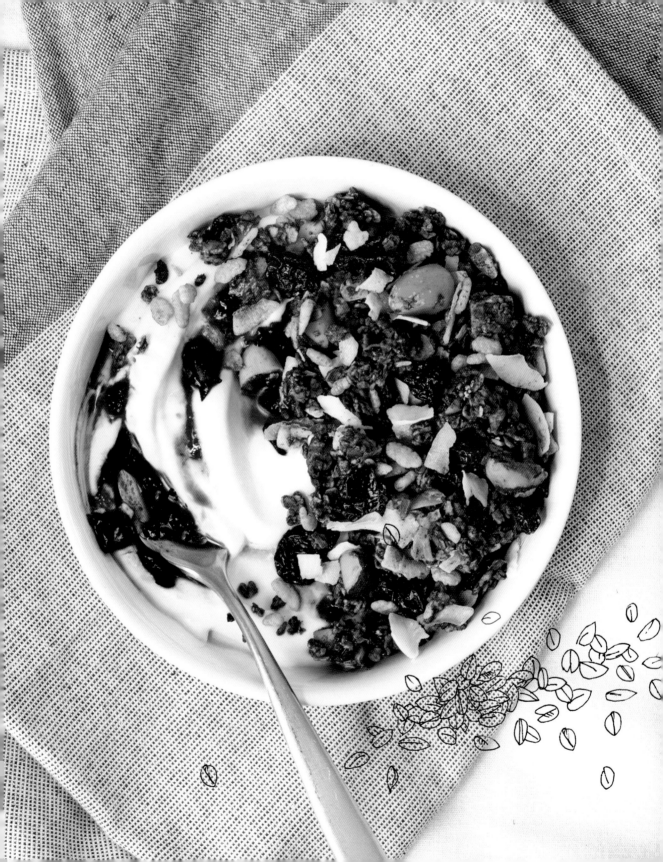

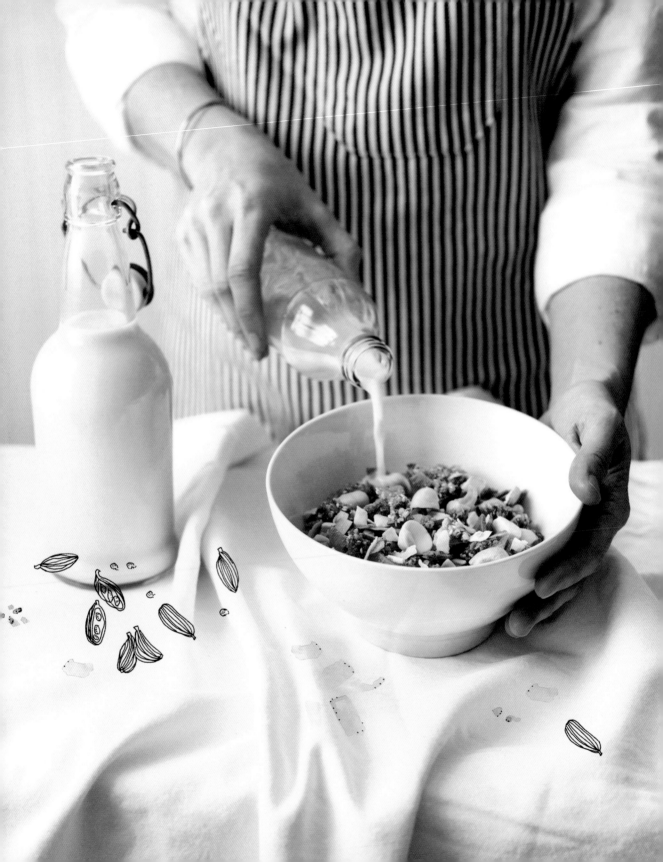

Coconut, Mango & Macadamia Granola

Need a vacation? Every bite of this flavorful, richly textured granola will take you far away. Try it with Coconut Yogurt (page 94), over a vanilla-bean Nice Cream (page 279), or by the handful for toes-in-the-sand daydreams. If you are ginger-crazed like me, try adding ½ cup (40 g) crystallized ginger pieces for extra spice and warmth.

SERVES 8+

1½ cups (120 g) rolled oats

1 cup (100 g) brown rice flakes

1 cup (240 ml) maple syrup

1 cup (135 g) raw or roasted macadamia nuts, chopped

½ cup (85 g) hulled buckwheat groats

¼ cup (60 ml) unrefined coconut oil

2 teaspoons grated orange zest

1 teaspoon grated lime zest

1 teaspoon peeled, grated fresh ginger—almost a pulp

1 teaspoon vanilla extract

¾ teaspoon sea salt

¼ teaspoon ground cardamom

1 cup (85 g) flaked coconut

½ cup (70 g) raw, unsalted cashews

1½ cups (175 g) dried mango, chopped or cut into pieces

1   Preheat the oven to 300°F (150°C). In a large bowl, combine the oats, brown rice flakes, maple syrup, macadamia nuts, buckwheat, coconut oil, zest, ginger, vanilla, salt, and cardamom. Spread the mixture on a rimmed baking sheet in an even layer roughly ¼ inch (6 mm) thick. Lightly press the mixture and bake for 20 minutes.

2   At the 20-minute mark, stir the coconut flakes and cashews into your granola until thoroughly incorporated. Lightly press down again and bake for 15 to 20 more minutes, until golden brown and well toasted. The granola continues baking once removed from the oven; let it cool and harden on the baking sheet.

3   Once cool, break apart the granola and fold in the dried mango. Store in an airtight container in the pantry or fridge for 4 to 8 weeks.

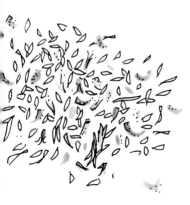

Earl Grey & Strawberry Granola

Black tea with the citrus burst of bergamot oil combines with vanilla and strawberry for a unique twist on starting the day. Look for rooibos-based Earl Grey tea if you want a decaf version. Serve with Coconut Yogurt (page 94), homemade Dairy-Free Milk (page 101), or some Nice Cream (page 279).

SERVES 8+

3 cups (240 g) rolled oats

1 cup (240 ml) raw, unpasteurized honey

¾ cup (105 g) raw, unsalted almonds, chopped

½ cup (70 g) raw, unsalted sunflower seeds

¼ cup (30 g) raw, unsalted pepitas

¼ cup (60 ml) extra virgin olive oil

1 tablespoon Earl Grey tea leaves, ground in coffee/spice grinder

1 teaspoon grated orange zest

¾ teaspoon sea salt

1 cup (20 g) dried strawberries

1. Preheat the oven to 300°F (150°C). In a large bowl, combine the oats, honey, almonds, sunflower seeds, pepitas, olive oil, tea, zest, and salt. Spread the mixture on a rimmed baking sheet in an even layer roughly ¼ inch (6 mm) thick. Give it a light press and bake for 35 to 40 minutes, stirring every 10 minutes, until toasty, golden brown.

2. Once cooled, transfer the granola to a large bowl and break apart; fold in the strawberries. Store in an airtight container in the pantry or fridge for 4 to 8 weeks.

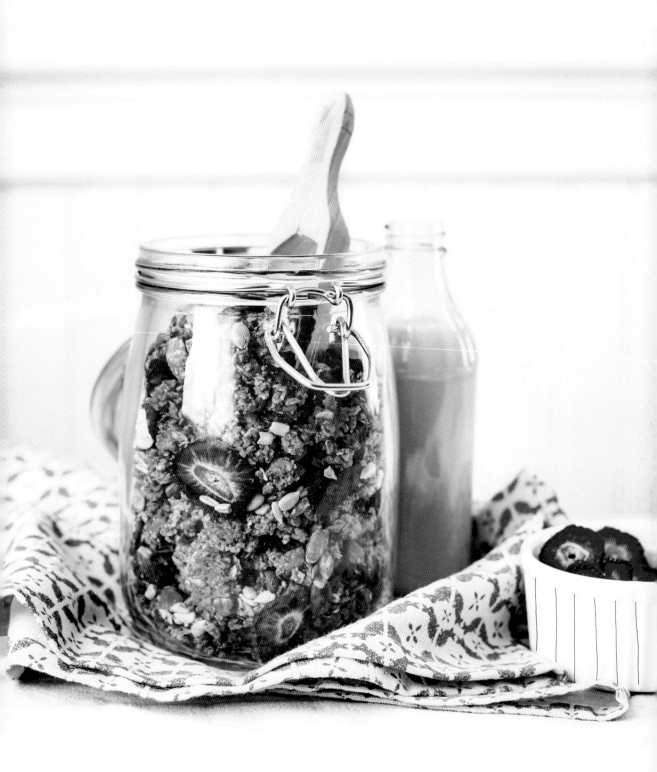

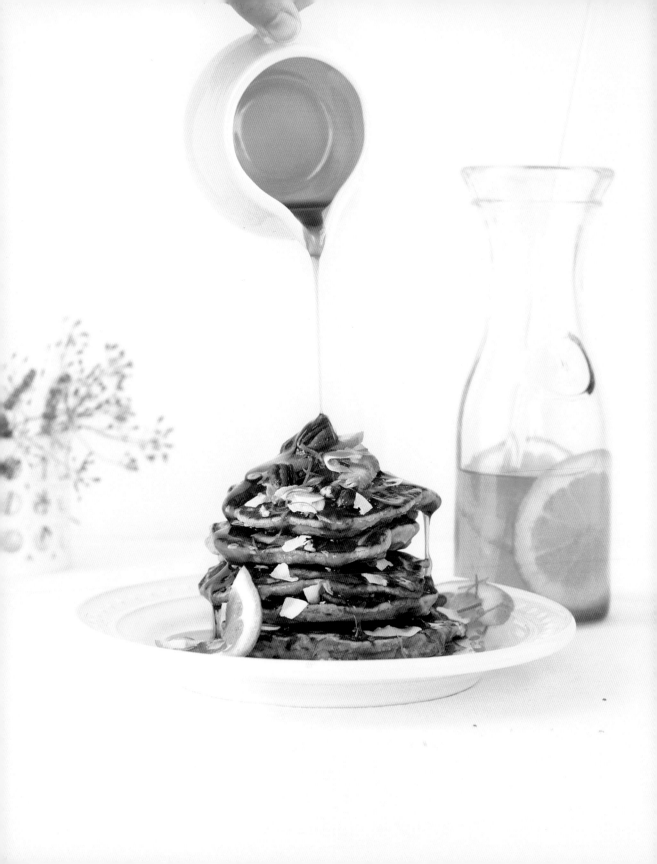

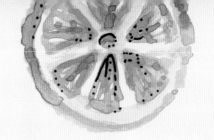
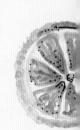

Pancakes & Waffles

Gluten-free pancakes don't have to taste like cardboard, and they don't have to be super involved either, unless you want them to be.

Make a big batch and freeze or pop in the fridge for future meals, with a sheet of parchment paper in between each so they don't stick together. Reheat in the toaster, oven, or a skillet, and enjoy them as snacks.

Serve with maple syrup, honey, jam, homemade fruit Compote (page 90), coconut cream, and/or nut butter. Make them savory and serve with spicy dips and veggies!

Pancake combo shown here:
Carrots, toasted pecans, toasted coconut & orange.

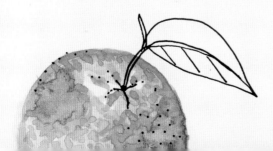

Pancakes & Waffles

4+ SERVINGS
COOK TIME: 15 TO 30 MINUTES

While there is a variety of gluten-free flours out there, this template shares the ratios and combinations that I find to be the most consistent when cooking, and most versatile when combined with Flavor and Fold-Ins. Note that bean flours are best for savory pancakes, which can be used to accompany curries and stews and are great for dipping!

What you need no matter what:

½ teaspoon baking powder

½ teaspoon baking soda

¼ teaspoon sea salt

1½ cups (360 ml) water, plus more if needed

1 to 2 tablespoon maple syrup or honey (only if making a sweet pancake)

1 In a large bowl, whisk together Flour, Binder, the **baking powder, baking soda,** and **salt.**

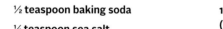

Flour ----- *and* -----> Binder

1½ CUPS TOTAL
Choose two or more

Brown rice flour

Garbanzo bean flour (best for savory pancakes)

Oat flour

Sorghum flour

Choose one

1¼ teaspoons whole psyllium husk

¾ teaspoon ground psyllium husk

½ ripe banana, mashed or blended (note: adds banana flavor)

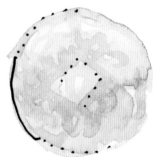

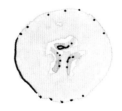

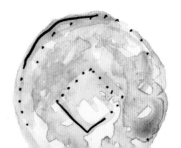

2 In another bowl, whisk together the **water, maple syrup or honey** (only if making a sweet pancake), and your Flavor (if using) until smooth. Fold into the dry ingredients, then gently whisk in the Fold-Ins (if using). Add more water, 1 tablespoon at a time, if needed to reach your favorite pancake batter consistency—should be like pouring a thick cream.

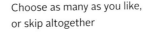

Flavor ---------- *and* --------→ **Fold-Ins**

Choose as many as you like, or skip altogether

Choose as many as you like, or skip altogether

¼ teaspoon ground cardamom

¼ teaspoon ground cinnamon

1 to 3 teaspoons grated citrus zest (orange, lemon, lime, tangerine, etc.)

1 to 2 teaspoons tea leaves (any), ground in coffee/spice grinder

1 teaspoon to 2 tablespoons fresh citrus juice (orange, lemon, lime, tangerine, etc.)

½ to 1 teaspoon ground ginger (or 1 to 2 teaspoons peeled, minced fresh ginger)

1 teaspoon extract (vanilla, almond, chocolate)

1 to 2 tablespoons natural sweetener (Sucanat; raw, unpasteurized honey; maple syrup)

2 to 4 tablespoons cacao nibs

1 to 3 tablespoons cocoa/cacao powder

¼ to ½ cup (45 to 90 g) chocolate chips

¼ to ½ cup (30 to 85 g) diced or shredded fruit (any)

¼ to ½ cup (35 to 70 g) nuts or large/medium seeds or 1 to 2 tablespoons small seeds like chia, poppy, or sesame

¼ cup (10 g) fresh herbs, chopped

¼ cup (20 g) shredded or flaked coconut

¼ to ½ cup (30 to 60 g) peeled, shredded raw veggies (root veg such as winter or summer squash)

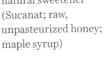

---

3 Heat a nonstick skillet or griddle over medium-high heat and add 1 teaspoon Oil to coat the bottom of the pan. (If using a waffle iron, grease with Oil and prepare to use according to the manufacturer's instructions.) Using a ladle, pour batter into the hot pan to create 4-inch (10 cm) pancakes or smaller silver dollars. When the edges of the pancakes are dry and the tops have bubbles, flip. Cook the other side for 2 to 3 minutes. Repeat, adding oil as necessary to the griddle, until all the batter is used. Serve sweet pancakes warm, topped with Compote (page 90), maple syrup, or honey, and savory pancakes with Fermented Veggies (page 153), Soups (page 175), or Hearty Chickpea Stew (page 183).

Oil Choose one

Unrefined coconut oil

Grapeseed oil

Sunflower seed oil

Avocado oil

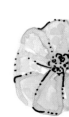

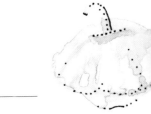

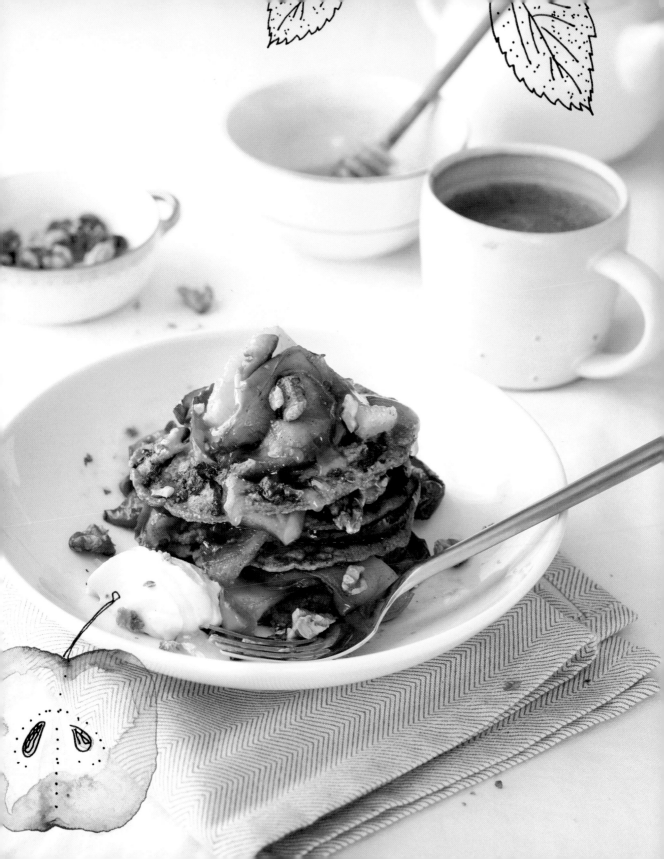

Beet Pancakes *with* Roasted Apples

What's more special than a pancake breakfast? A pink pancake breakfast. Add a dollop of Coconut Yogurt (page 94) or coconut cream (from a chilled can of coconut milk) to top these pancakes.

SERVES 4+

4 red apples, cored and sliced (peels on or off—chef's choice)

1 large orange (any kind)

¼ cup (60 ml) unrefined coconut oil, gently warmed to liquid, plus more if needed

¼ cup (60 ml) raw, unpasteurized honey, gently warmed over low heat, plus more if needed

1 teaspoon ground cinnamon

½ teaspoon ground cardamom

Pinch plus ¼ teaspoon sea salt

½ cup (80 g) brown rice flour

½ cup (50 g) oat flour

½ cup (60 g) sorghum flour

¾ teaspoon ground psyllium husk

½ teaspoon baking powder

½ teaspoon baking soda

1½ cups (360 ml) water, plus more if needed

1 teaspoon vanilla extract

½ cup (70 g; about 1 small) peeled, shredded beet

½ cup (50 g) walnuts, toasted and chopped

1. Preheat the oven to 400°F (200°C) and scatter the apples into a glass baking dish.

2. Supreme the orange (remove the peel and membranes), setting the wedges aside and reserving 1 tablespoon juice. Pour the juice over the apples, then drizzle 2 tablespoons coconut oil over them, following with 3 tablespoons honey. Sprinkle the apples with the cinnamon, ¼ teaspoon cardamom, and a pinch of salt. Roast for 15 to 20 minutes, shaking at the 5- and 10-minute marks. Remove from the oven, cover, and set aside.

3. In a large bowl, whisk together the flours, remaining cardamom and sea salt, the psyllium, baking powder, and baking soda until thoroughly mixed.

4. In another bowl, whisk together the water, remaining honey, and vanilla until smooth, then fold in the dry ingredients and beet. Add more water, 1 tablespoon at a time, until the batter is like pourable cream.

5. Heat a nonstick skillet or griddle over medium heat and add 1 teaspoon coconut oil. Use a ladle to pour batter into 3- to 4-inch (7.5 to 10 cm) pancakes. When the edges of the pancakes dry and the tops bubble, flip. Cook the other side for 2 to 3 minutes. Repeat, adding more oil if necessary. Layer the pancakes with the orange wedges, apples, honey, and walnuts.

Meyer Lemon Waffles *with* Maple-Blackberry Compote

When I get my hands on Meyer lemons, my inner schoolgirl squeals! Their sweet, floral flavor makes this recipe special—you'll need one large Meyer lemon (or two small). Can't find Meyer lemons? Regular lemons work fine. No waffle iron? Make pancakes instead.

MAKES 8 WAFFLES

Maple-Blackberry Compote
(from page 90 template)

3 cups (435 g) blackberries

1 teaspoon lemon juice

¼ cup (60 ml) maple syrup

—

Toasted Coconut Cream
(optional)

One 13.5-ounce (400 ml) can
full-fat coconut milk, chilled

¼ cup (20 g) flaked
coconut, toasted

Meyer Lemon Waffles

Unrefined coconut oil

½ cup (80 g) brown rice flour

½ cup (50 g) oat flour

½ cup (60 g) sorghum flour

¾ teaspoon ground psyllium husk

½ teaspoon baking powder

½ teaspoon baking soda

¼ teaspoon sea salt

1½ cups (360 ml) water

2 tablespoons Meyer lemon juice

2 teaspoons grated Meyer
lemon zest

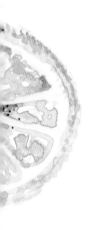

1. Follow the simple steps on page 91 to prepare the Maple-Blackberry Compote. If making the Toasted Coconut Cream, open the can of chilled coconut milk. Scoop out the solid cream on top and transfer to a large bowl—save the liquid in the fridge for Soup (page 175) or a smoothie. Whisk together the toasted coconut and cream and place in the fridge to chill.

2. Preheat a waffle iron and grease with oil.

3. In a large bowl, whisk together the flours, psyllium, baking powder, baking soda, and salt until thoroughly mixed.

4. In another bowl, whisk together the water and lemon juice. Fold together with the dry ingredients and then incorporate the zest.

5. Using a ladle, pour batter into the waffle iron and cook until the edges are crispy. Repeat, adding more oil when necessary, until all batter is used. Top with Maple-Blackberry Compote and a dollop of Toasted Coconut Cream.

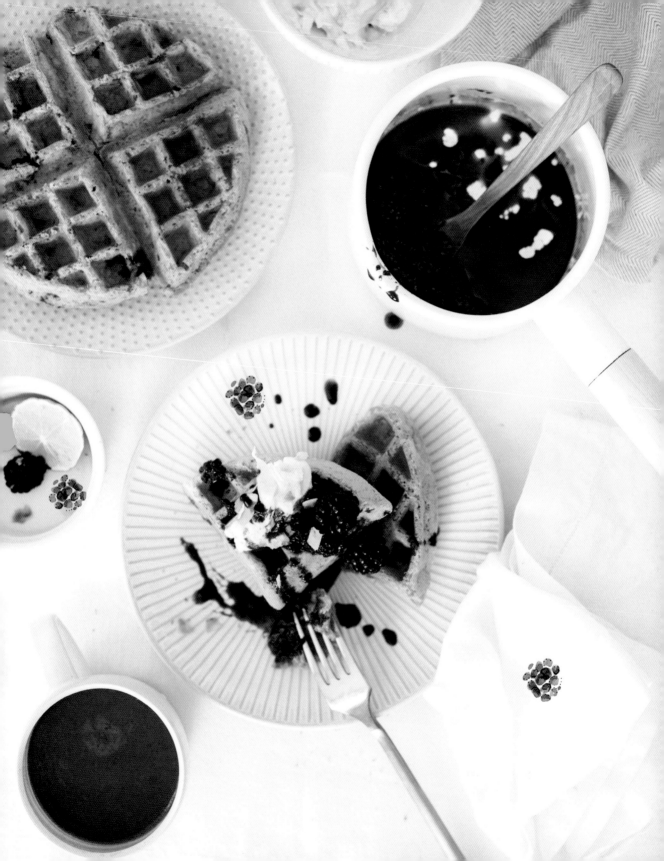

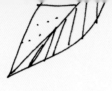

Cashew-Coconut Buttercream

Transform muffins into cupcakes with this decadent frosting. Simply blend together all ingredients until ultra-creamy and chill until firm. Spread or pipe onto cooled or chilled muffins.

½ cup (70 g) cashews, soaked for 12 hours for maximum plumpness

1 cup (220 g) coconut cream from top of can of chilled coconut milk (about 2 cans' worth)

3 tablespoons raw honey or maple syrup

2 tablespoons unrefined coconut oil

1 teaspoon apple cider vinegar

1 teaspoon vanilla extract

¼ teaspoon sea salt

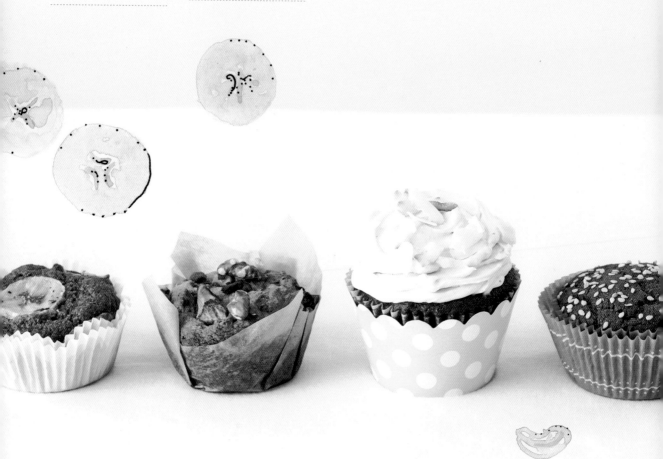

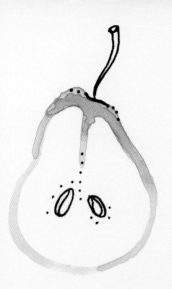

Muffins

You don't need me to tell you that finding a delicious gluten-free muffin without suspicious gums or excessive starches can be quite the challenge. After years of playing and fine-tuning, I can share with you my favorite template for incredible muffins you can feel great about—sweet and savory.

Use a savory muffin for dunking into Soups (page 175) and Hearty Chickpea Stew (page 183). Crumble leftover sweetened muffins into a greased baking dish, fold in some chopped fruit, pour some coconut cream on top, and bake for bread pudding. Play.

Muffin combos shown here from left to right:
Banana-almond; Savory Olive Oil, Zucchini & Walnut (page 68);
vanilla bean with Cashew-Coconut Buttercream (opposite),
toasted sesame & orange; Classic Blueberry (page 71).

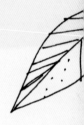

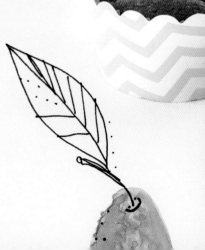

Muffins

MAKES 8 TO 10
BAKE TIME: 30 MINUTES

I call for blanched almond flour in this template because it bakes up light and cakey. I also call for arrowroot to add a nice crumb to the muffin texture, but you can leave it out.

Store muffins in the fridge in an airtight glass container for 7 to 14 days. Freeze for up to two months. The binders in this recipe work—substitute with anything not listed at your own risk!

What you need no matter what:

¾ cup (85 g) blanched almond flour

¼ cup (30 g) arrowroot flour/starch

1½ teaspoons baking soda

1 teaspoon baking powder

¼ teaspoon sea salt

¾ cup (180 ml) warm water

1 Preheat the oven to 350°F (180°C) and line a muffin pan with unbleached parchment-paper liners. Then, in a large bowl, sift together Grain Flour, Spice (if using), and Sweet plus the **almond flour, arrowroot, baking soda, baking powder,** and **salt.**

Grain Flour 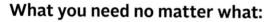 *and/or* ⟶ Spice

1 CUP TOTAL
Choose one or combine

Oat flour

Sorghum flour

Gluten-free all-purpose flour

Choose one or combine, or skip altogether

½ to 1 teaspoon ground cinnamon

¼ teaspoon ground cardamom

2 tablespoons pumpkin pie spice

3 tablespoons cocoa/cacao powder

Pinch to ¼ teaspoon ground cloves

Pinch to ¼ teaspoon fresh-ground nutmeg

Sweet

1 CUP (200 G)
Choose one or combine; skip for a savory muffin, but add another ½ cup Grain Flour in its place

Sucanat

Rapadura

Coconut sugar

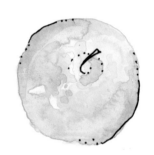

2 In another bowl, mix the **warm water** with Purée, Flavor (if using), Oil, and Acid.

Purée ············ *and/or* ············→ Flavor

½ CUP TOTAL
Choose one or combine; purée adding
1 to 2 tablespoons of water if needed

Apple (any kind) or applesauce	Beets (any kind), steamed	Pumpkin, steamed
Pear (any kind)	Butternut squash, steamed	Sweet potato, steamed
Banana		

Choose one or combine, or skip altogether

1 teaspoon extract (vanilla, almond, cocoa, hazelnut)

1 to 4 teaspoons peeled, minced fresh ginger

1 to 3 teaspoons grated citrus zest

Oil ················· *and* ················→ Acid

3 TABLESPOONS TOTAL
Choose one or combine

Extra virgin olive oil (tasty with citrus like orange and lemon; great for a savory muffin)

Unrefined coconut oil

Grapeseed oil

1 TABLESPOON
Choose one or combine

Apple cider vinegar

Fresh lemon juice

Fresh lime juice

---

3 If using psyllium as your Binder, whisk it into the dry ingredients until thoroughly incorporated. If using banana as your Binder, mix it into the wet ingredients. Mix the wet and dry ingredients together and incorporate Fold-Ins (if using). Spoon batter into the parchment-lined muffin pan, filling each cup three-quarters full. Bake for 30 to 35 minutes, until the tops and edges are dry and browned. Remove and cool in the pan.

Binder ············ *and/or* ············→ Fold-Ins

Choose one

2 teaspoons whole psyllium husk

1½ teaspoons ground psyllium husk

1 ripe banana, mashed or blended (adds banana flavor and sweetness)

½ TO ¾ CUP TOTAL
Choose one or combine, or skip altogether

Pome fruit (any kind), cored and diced

Banana, diced

Berries (any kind)

Coconut, shredded or flaked

Stone fruit/dates (any kind), pitted

Chocolate chips

Summer or winter squash, diced

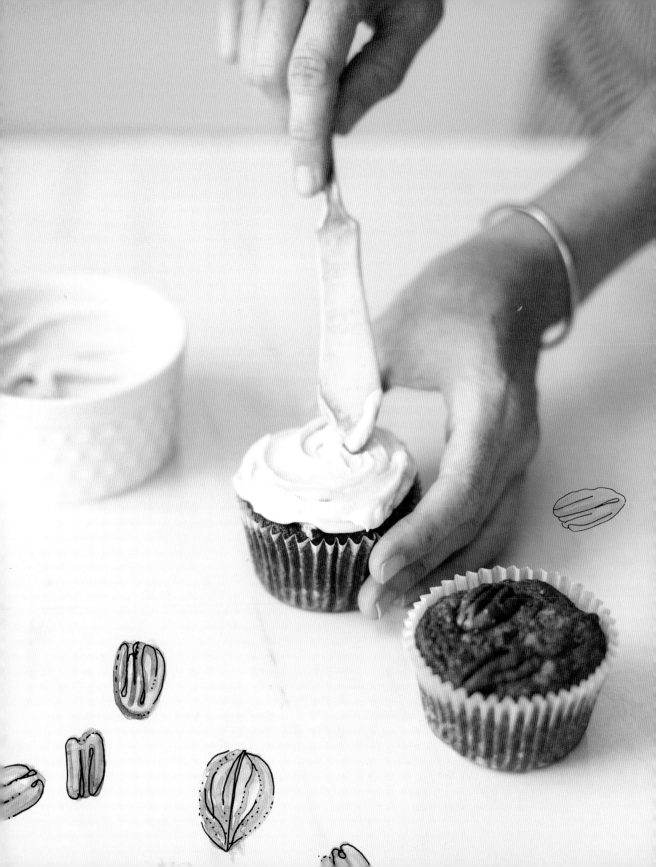

Sweet Potato Muffins

This is a recipe that I've made for years for family—I've had great intentions to share on YumUniverse.com but never got around to it. I'm glad I waited, because it's special and deserves to be in print.

MAKES 12+ MUFFINS

1 to 2 large sweet potatoes (½ cup/100 g diced, plus ½ cup/160 g shredded), peeled or unpeeled

½ cup (50 g) raw, unsalted pecans

Pinch plus ¼ teaspoon sea salt

1 cup (200 g) Sucanat

1 cup (120 g) sorghum flour

¾ cup (85 g) blanched almond flour

¼ cup (30 g) arrowroot starch/flour

1½ teaspoons baking soda

1½ teaspoons ground psyllium husk

1 teaspoon baking powder

1 teaspoon ground cinnamon

½ teaspoon fresh-ground nutmeg

Pinch ground cloves

¾ cup (180 ml) warm water

3 tablespoons unrefined coconut oil

1 tablespoon fresh lemon juice

1 tablespoon peeled, minced fresh ginger— almost a pulp

1 teaspoon vanilla extract

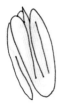

1 Preheat the oven to 350°F (180°C). Steam the diced sweet potato for 20 to 35 minutes, until soft and easily pierced with a fork. Blend or mash (with 1 to 2 tablespoons of water if necessary) until you get a purée. Transfer to a large bowl and set aside.

2 Line a muffin pan with unbleached parchment liners and also line a baking sheet with unbleached parchment paper. Spread the pecans in a layer on the baking sheet, sprinkle with a pinch of salt, and pop in the oven for 7 minutes. Remove, chop, and set aside.

3 In a large bowl, sift together the Sucanat, flours, baking soda, psyllium husk, baking powder, remaining ¼ teaspoon salt, cinnamon, nutmeg, and cloves.

4 In the large bowl with the sweet potato purée, whisk in the water, coconut oil, lemon juice, ginger, and vanilla extract. Gently fold into the dry ingredients and then incorporate the shredded sweet potato and toasted pecans until well mixed. Spoon batter into the parchment-lined muffin cups until each is three-quarters full. Bake for 30 minutes, or until the tops and edges are dry and browned. Remove and cool in the pan.

Savory Olive Oil, Zucchini & Walnut Muffins

You can make a savory muffin simply by following the template, making savory choices and omitting the Sweet in Step 1. These muffins are delicious served warm with a spread of coconut oil and/or honey and make a great substitute for dinner rolls, too. Enjoy them with Hearty Chickpea Stew (page 183).

MAKES 12+ MUFFINS

¼ cup (25 g) raw, unsalted walnuts, chopped

Pinch plus ¼ teaspoon sea salt

1 cup (105 g) oat flour

¾ cup (85 g) blanched almond flour

1½ teaspoons baking soda

1½ teaspoons ground psyllium husk

1 teaspoon baking powder

¾ cup (180 ml) warm water

½ cup (120 g) applesauce

3 tablespoons extra virgin olive oil

1 tablespoon fresh lemon juice

¾ cup (95 g) shredded zucchini

½ cup (90 g) Cashew-Almond Cheese Crumbles (optional, page 133) or store-bought firm, plant-based cheese grated or crumbled

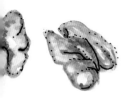

1   Preheat the oven to 350°F (180°C). Line a muffin pan with unbleached parchment liners. Also line a baking sheet with unbleached parchment paper and spread the walnuts into one layer on the sheet. Sprinkle with a pinch of salt and pop in the oven for 7 minutes. Remove, chop, and set aside.

2   In a large bowl, sift together the flours, baking soda, psyllium husk, baking powder, and remaining ¼ teaspoon salt.

3   In another large bowl, whisk together the water, applesauce, oil, and lemon juice. Gently fold into the dry ingredients and then incorporate the zucchini, toasted walnuts, and Cashew-Almond Cheese Crumbles (if using) until well mixed.

4   Spoon batter into the parchment-lined muffin cups until each is three-quarters full. Bake for 30 minutes, or until the tops and edges are dry and browned. Remove and cool in the pan.

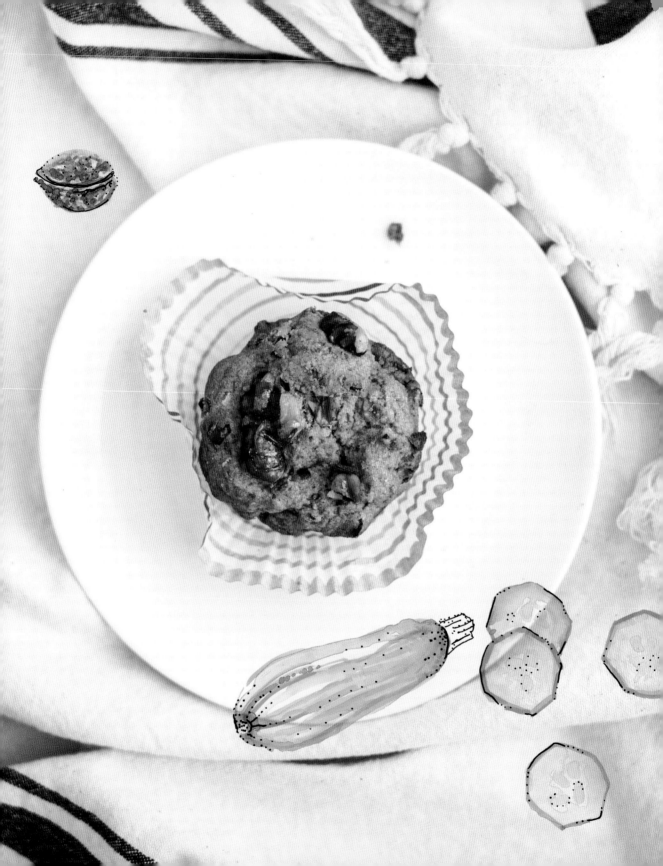

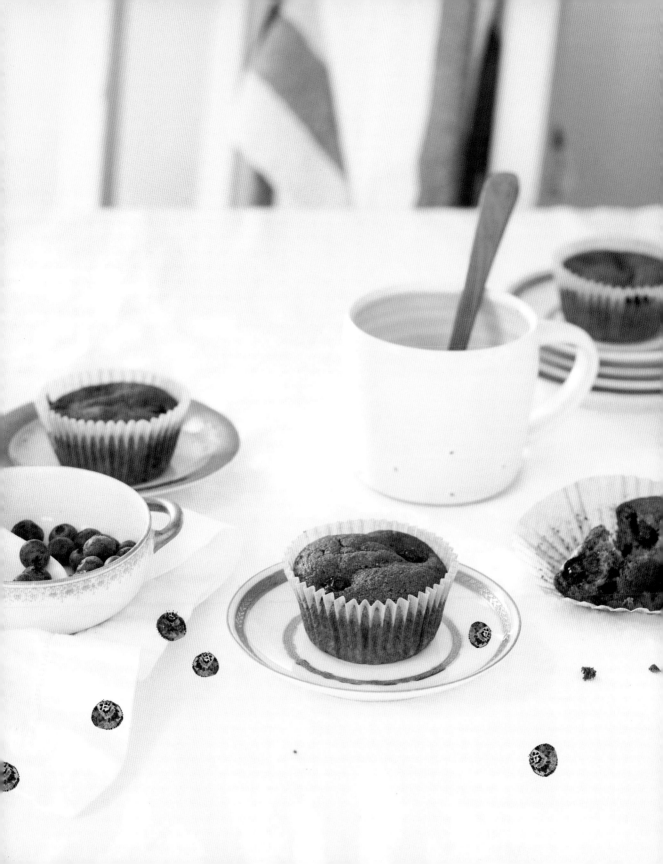

Classic Blueberry Muffins

When I was a girl, I only ate white foods. No veggies, no fruit.
On weekends, my father used to make the most beautiful blueberry
muffins for my little brother and me—loaded with ginormous,
juicy blueberries. But berries were blue. And fruit. So, I would pick
them out one by one and hand them over to Dad to eat. I look back and
shake my head at the blasphemy of it all. This one's for you, Dad.

MAKES 12+ MUFFINS

1 cup (200 g) coconut sugar

1 cup (105 g) oat flour

¾ cup (85 g) blanched
almond flour

¼ cup (30 g) arrowroot
starch/flour

1½ teaspoons baking soda

1½ teaspoons ground
psyllium husk

1 teaspoon baking powder

¼ teaspoon sea salt

¾ cup (180 ml) warm water

½ cup (120 g) applesauce

3 tablespoons unrefined
coconut oil

1 tablespoon fresh lemon juice

1 teaspoon vanilla extract

½ cup (70 g) fresh blueberries
(in a pinch you can use frozen,
thawed berries)

1. Preheat the oven to 350°F (180°C). Line a muffin pan with unbleached parchment liners and set aside.

2. In a large bowl, sift together the sugar, all the flours, baking soda, psyllium husk, baking powder, and salt.

3. In another large bowl, whisk together the water, applesauce, coconut oil, lemon juice, and vanilla extract. Gently fold into the dry ingredients and incorporate the blueberries until well mixed.

4. Spoon batter into the parchment-lined muffin pan cups until each is three-quarters full. Bake for 35 minutes, or until the tops and edges are dry and browned. Remove and cool in the pan.

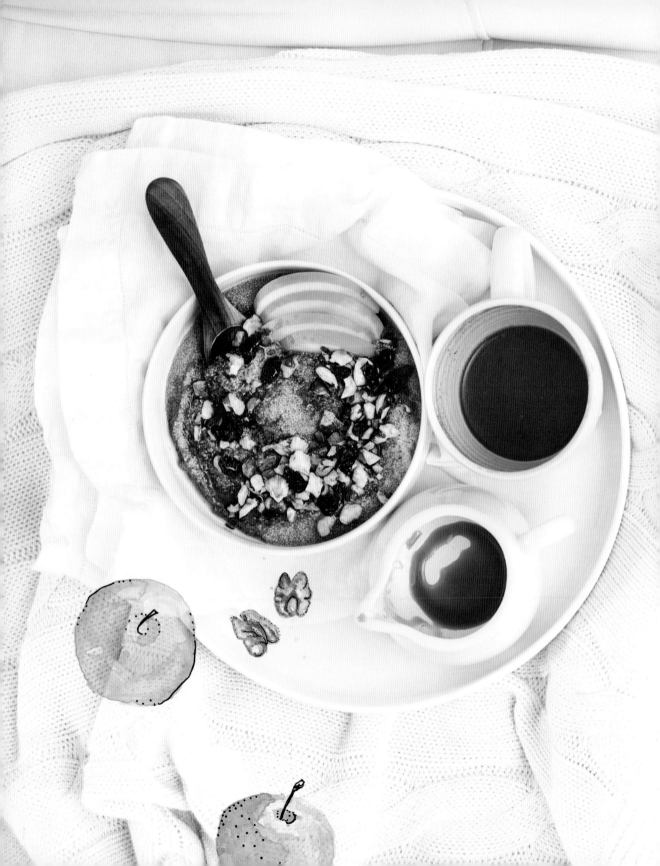

Warm Cereals

As a kiddo, I loved warm Cream of Wheat
(with a mountain of sugar on top) drowned in cold milk.
It was, after all, in my beloved sugary-white-foods group.

As an adult, I can tap into that comforting childhood
nostalgia while completely avoiding the gluten and
dreaded sugar crash. You can pull from a colorful palette of
nutrient-rich grains, nuts, seeds, toppings, spices, and
fruit to whip up something for a simple food mood, or
you can get fancy-pants with unique ingredients, heirloom
fruits, and creative additions like ground tea,
exotic spices, and herbs.

Oh! You can also bake warm cereal (with a touch of
extra Sweet) in ramekins for a rice-pudding-style dessert.
So many options.

Warm Cereal combo shown here: Cacao-maple-cinnamon amaranth & teff swirl
with toasted walnuts, goji berries & Granny Smith apple.

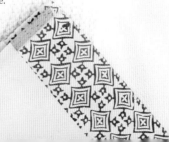

Warm Cereals

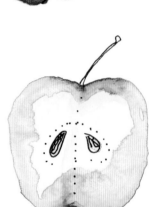

2+ SERVINGS
COOK TIME: 5 TO 7 MINUTES

Do yourself a solid and prepare a little bit. Soak and cook cereal grains in advance (see page 11) and store until ready to use in an airtight glass container in the fridge for a week or two, or the freezer for a month or more. Use frozen fruit in a pinch, and a simple combo of water and nut butter stirred directly into the cereal when Dairy-Free Milk isn't on hand (to make your own, see page 101).

What you need no matter what:

1 to 2 teaspoons unrefined coconut oil (optional)   ¼ teaspoon sea salt

1 In a pot heated to medium, stir together Cereal Grains, ½ cup (120 ml) Dairy-Free Milk, and, if you like, the **oil** and stir for 1 minute. Add more milk, ¼ cup (60 ml) at a time, to reach your preferred taste and consistency.

Cereal Grains ----- *and* ---→ Dairy-Free Milk

1½ CUPS TOTAL
Choose one or combine; page 11 for cooking tips

Amaranth, cooked

Black forbidden rice, cooked

Brown rice, cooked

Buckwheat, cooked

Millet, cooked

Quick rolled oats, uncooked

Polenta, cooked

Quinoa, cooked

Teff (any kind), cooked

½ TO 1½ CUPS (120 TO 240 ML) TOTAL
Choose one

Almond milk

Brown rice milk

Coconut milk

Cashew milk

Macadamia milk

Pecan milk

Walnut milk

Sunflower seed milk

Oat milk

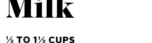
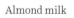
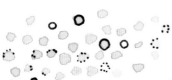

2 Stir together Flavor, Fun Additions (if using), and/or Sweet (if using), and the **salt** and cook for 3 to 5 minutes more.

Flavor ············· *and* ············→ Fun Additions

Choose one or combine

Choose one or combine, or skip altogether

1 to 2 tablespoons cacao nibs	¼ teaspoon ground cloves	1 to 2 tablespoons cocoa/cacao powder
Pinch to ¼ teaspoon ground cardamom	¼ teaspoon ground nutmeg	2 tablespoons ground coffee
Pinch to ¼ teaspoon cayenne pepper	¼ to 1 teaspoon extract (almond, chocolate, hazelnut, vanilla)	1 teaspoon fennel seed
1 to 2 teaspoons ground cinnamon	¼ to 1 teaspoon grated citrus zest	½ to 1 teaspoon ground ginger (or 1 to 2 teaspoons peeled, minced fresh ginger)
1 to 2 teaspoons pumpkin pie spice	1 to 3 teaspoons fresh citrus juice	

¼ to ½ teaspoon tea leaves, ground in coffee/spice grinder (black, chai, chicory root, dandelion root, Earl Grey, rooibos, matcha, chamomile)

1 to 4 teaspoons fresh herbs (thyme, lavender, basil, mint, tarragon)

¼ cup diced or shredded winter squash or root veggies, roasted or steamed

1 to 2 tablespoons unsalted nut or seed butter

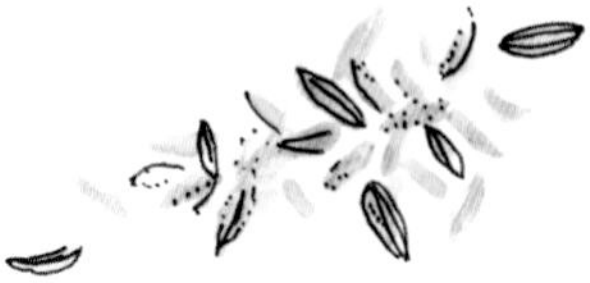

Sweet

Choose one or combine, or skip altogether

1 to 2 tablespoons maple syrup	1 to 2 tablespoons raw, unpasteurized honey	1 to 2 tablespoons Sucanat
		1 to 2 tablespoons brown rice syrup

1 to 2 tablespoons coconut sugar

1 to 2 tablespoons blackstrap molasses

---

3 Spoon into a serving bowl, add Toppings (if using), and enjoy warm.

Toppings

Choose one or combine, or skip altogether

¼ to 1 cup fresh or dried fruit (pome, stone, berries, tropical, raisins, pitted dates, pomegranate)

¼ to ½ cup (20 to 45 g) toasted coconut, flaked or shredded

¼ to ½ cup (35 to 70 g) chopped nuts and/or seeds, toasted

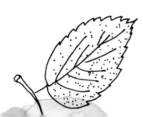

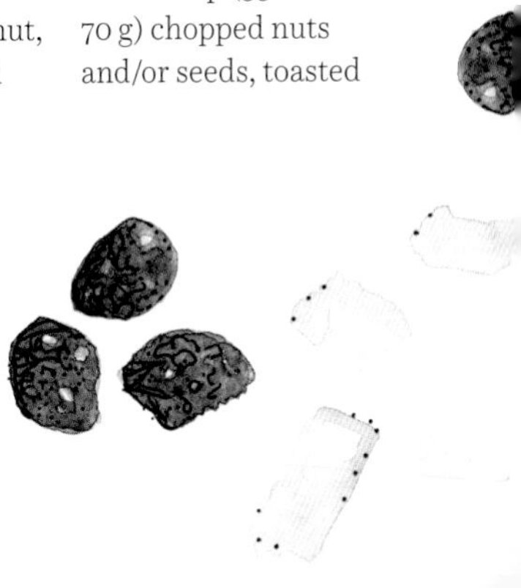

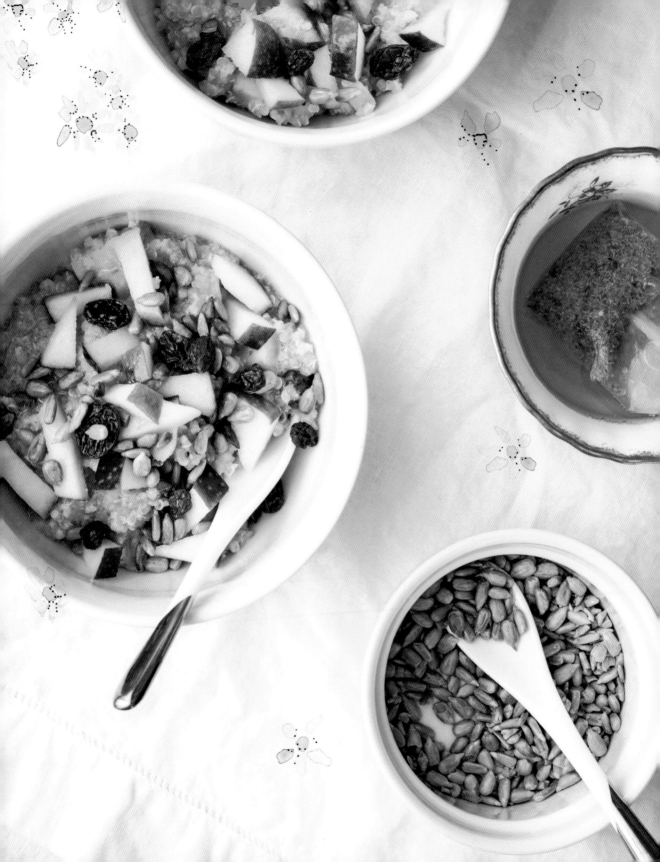

Chamomile, Apple & Ancient Grain Bowl

I love tea and have multiple drawers in my kitchen dedicated to a variety of them. When I can, I add some to my cooking and baking for unique flavor. This recipe calls for tea ground into a powder, but if you don't have the tools for this step, simply use steeped tea (2 to 3 bags for deep flavor) as your cooking water when preparing your grains—it will infuse them beautifully.

SERVES 1+

¼ cup (35 g) raw, unsalted sunflower seeds

Pinch plus ¼ teaspoon sea salt, plus more to taste

1 red apple (any kind)

2 teaspoons fresh lemon juice

1 cup (240 ml) canned coconut milk

¼ cup (60 g) cooked amaranth (2 to 3 tablespoons dry, see page 11)

½ cup (85 g) cooked millet (3 tablespoons dry, see page 11)

½ cup (90 g) cooked quinoa (3 tablespoons dry, see page 11)

1 teaspoon unrefined coconut oil

½ teaspoon chamomile tea flowers, ground in coffee/spice grinder

1 tablespoon raw, unpasteurized honey

½ teaspoon vanilla extract

¼ cup (35 g) golden raisins

2 teaspoons chia seeds

1. Preheat the oven to 350°F (180°C). Line a baking sheet with unbleached parchment paper and spread sunflower seeds in a single layer on the sheet with room to roast mostly untouched on all sides. Sprinkle with a pinch of salt and pop in the oven for 7 minutes. Remove and set aside.

2. Core and dice (or slice) your apple, then toss with 1 teaspoon of the lemon juice—set aside.

3. In a large saucepan or pot heated to medium, stir together the milk, amaranth, millet, quinoa, and oil and stir for 1 minute. Add the remaining 1 teaspoon lemon juice, tea, honey, and remaining ¼ teaspoon salt; stir for 3 to 5 minutes more.

4. Spoon the warm cereal into a serving bowl, stir in the apple, raisins, and chia seeds, then sprinkle with the toasted sunflower seeds. Enjoy warm.

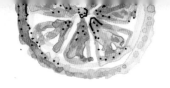

Ginger, Molasses & Date Oatmeal *with* Toasted Almonds

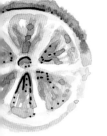

I pretty much make it through the winter on this combination—warming ginger, comforting, iron-rich molasses, and caramel-y dates are just the thing for a chilly morning. Great with apples, pears, and steamed winter squash, too.

SERVES 2+

1 navel orange

¼ cup (35 g) raw, unsalted almonds

Pinch plus ¼ teaspoon sea salt, plus more to taste

1½ cups (360 ml) almond milk

1½ cups (120 g) quick-cooking oats

1 teaspoon unrefined coconut oil

2 tablespoons blackstrap molasses, plus more for drizzle

2 teaspoons peeled, minced fresh ginger—almost a pulp

½ teaspoon ground cinnamon

½ teaspoon vanilla extract

¼ teaspoon ground cloves

¼ cup (35 g) pitted and chopped dates (any kind)

1 Supreme the orange (remove the peel and membrane from the fruit) and chop if you like; set aside.

2 Preheat the oven to 350°F (180°C). Line a baking sheet with unbleached parchment paper and spread the almonds in a single layer on the sheet with room to roast mostly untouched on all sides. Sprinkle with a pinch of salt and pop in the oven for 7 minutes. Remove, chop, and set aside.

3 In a large saucepan or pot heated to medium, stir together the milk, oats, and oil and cook for 1 minute. Add the molasses, ginger, cinnamon, vanilla extract, cloves, and remaining ¼ teaspoon salt; stir for 5 minutes more.

4 Spoon the warm cereal into a serving bowl, stir in the dates, sprinkle with the toasted almonds and orange—drizzle with more molasses if you like. Enjoy warm.

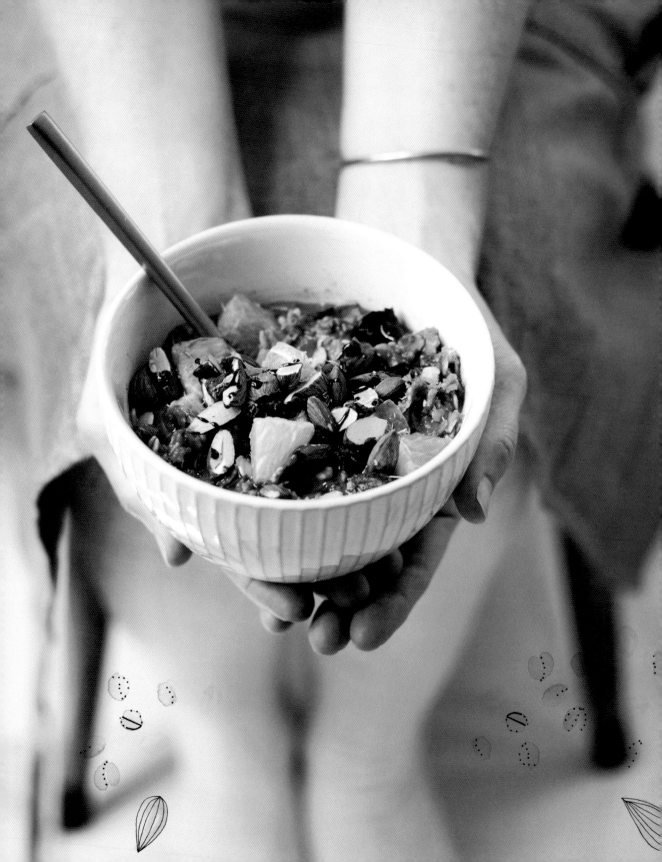

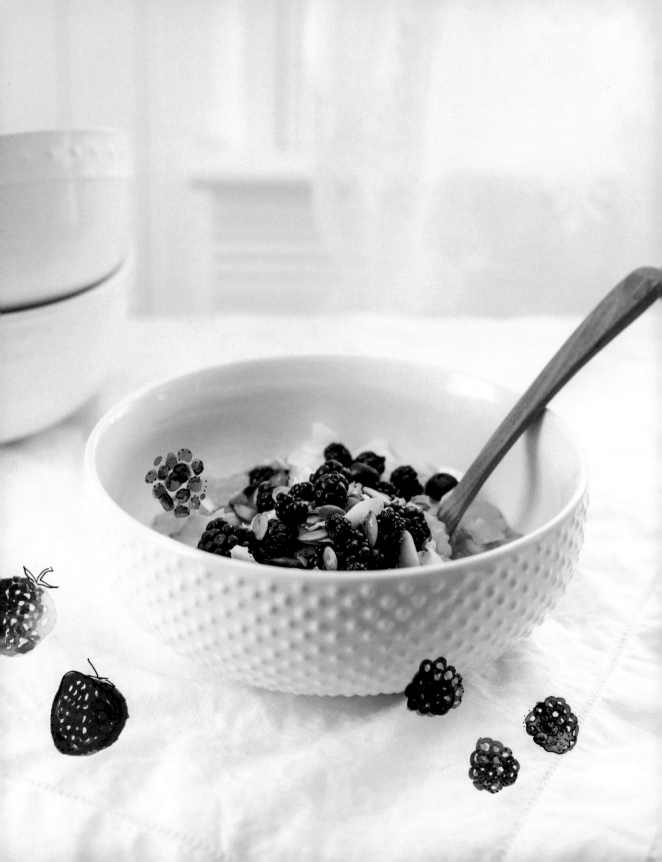

Breakfast Polenta *with* Mixed Berries & Salted Pepitas

If you like grits, you'll love this recipe since both are made from stone-ground cornmeal. I sometimes skip the honey and let the sweetness come only from the juicy berries, so do the same if you want it more on the savory side.

SERVES 1+

¼ cup (35 g) raw, unsalted pepitas

Pinch plus ¼ teaspoon sea salt, plus more to taste

¼ cup (20 g) dried coconut flakes

1½ cups (350 g) cooked polenta (½ cup/70 g dry)

1 cup (240 ml) coconut milk (canned or beverage style)

2 teaspoons unrefined coconut oil

2 teaspoons fresh lime juice

1 teaspoon grated lime zest

1 to 2 tablespoons raw, unpasteurized honey, to taste

¼ teaspoon cayenne pepper

1 cup (140 g) mixed berries (any kind)

1. Preheat the oven to 350°F (180°C). Line a baking sheet with unbleached parchment paper and spread the pepitas in one layer on the sheet so they have room to toast mostly untouched on all sides. Sprinkle with the pinch of salt and pop in the oven for 7 minutes. Remove from the baking sheet and set aside in a bowl.

2. Spread the coconut flakes onto the parchment-lined sheet and toast in the oven for 2 to 3 minutes—keep your eye on it so it doesn't burn. Set aside with the pepitas.

3. In a large saucepan or pot heated to medium, stir together the cooked polenta (either crumbled, cut into chunks, or creamy), coconut milk, and coconut oil; stir for 1 minute. Add the lime juice and zest, honey to taste, remaining ¼ teaspoon salt, and cayenne; stir for 3 to 5 minutes more.

4. Spoon the warm cereal into a serving bowl, load it up with fresh berries, then sprinkle with the toasted pepitas and flaked coconut. Enjoy warm.

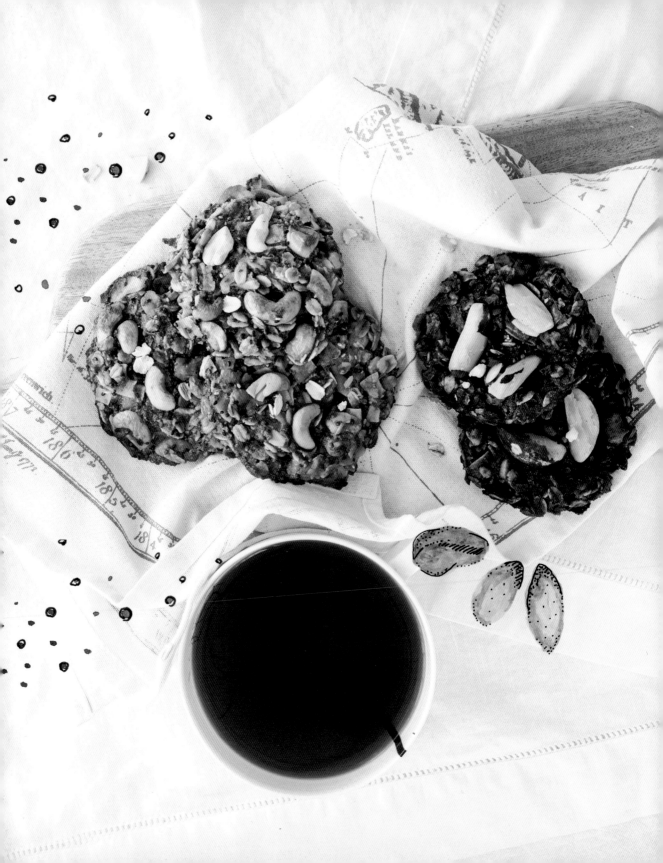

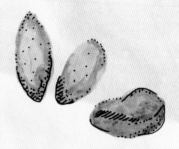

Breakfast Cookies

Breakfast cookies (a.k.a. everything-but-the-kitchen-sink cookies) are the best because, hey, it's cookies for breakfast, and also because it's grab-and-go food you can feel great about. Customize with countless combinations of nuts, seeds, spices, and fruit.

Take them to the office, on road trips, on planes—just keep a few with you so you aren't stuck somewhere without a satisfying, healthful snack.

Breakfast Cookie combos on this spread from left to right:
Chia, orange & cashew; cacao, coconut, coffee & Brazil nut.

Breakfast Cookies

MAKES 12 TO 14
COOK TIME: 15 TO 20 MINUTES

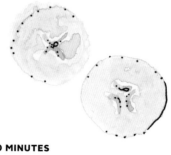

A comforting bowl of oatmeal in cookie form. For extra flavor, toast coconut, nuts, and seeds before mixing. When adding Flavor and Sweet, start with less and add more to taste before baking.

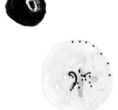

What you need no matter what:

1 cup (80 g) rolled oats, uncooked

½ teaspoon sea salt

¼ cup (60 ml) dairy-free milk or water, gently warmed

2 tablespoons unrefined coconut oil, gently warmed to liquid

1 Preheat the oven to 350°F (180°C). In a large bowl, combine the **oats** with Nuts & Seeds, Teenies (if using), **salt,** Dry Sweet (if using), and Binder (sprinkle it all over the mixture so it incorporates evenly). Stir until well mixed.

Nuts & Seeds ---- *and/or* → Teenies

½ CUP TOTAL
Choose one or combine; raw, unsalted; toast at 350°F (180°C) for 7 to 10 minutes for extra flavor; chop into small pieces

Almonds	Hazelnuts	Pine nuts
Brazil nuts	Pecans	Sunflower seeds
Cashews	Pepitas	Walnuts

1 TO 2 TABLESPOONS
Choose one or combine or skip altogether; start with raw and toast poppy or sesame for extra flavor

| Poppy seeds | Sesame seeds |
| Chia seeds | |

Dry Sweet --------- *and* --------→ Binder

2 TABLESPOONS TOTAL
Choose one or skip altogether

| Coconut sugar | Rapadura |
| Sucanat | |

Choose one

| 1 teaspoon whole psyllium husk | ½ teaspoon ground psyllium husk |

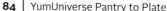

2 Add Flavor (if using) to the dry ingredients and mix well. In a small bowl, stir together Moisture, Sticky Sweet, warm **dairy-free milk or water,** and warm **coconut oil** until well mixed. Fold together the wet and dry ingredients and then stir in Texture.

Flavor Optional

*Choose any of these in combination **AND/OR** ----------------> *Choose one of these by itself*

2 to 4 tablespoons cacao nibs

¼ teaspoon ground cardamom

¼ teaspoon cayenne pepper

1 to 2 teaspoons ground cinnamon

¼ teaspoon ground cloves

¼ teaspoon ground nutmeg

½ to 1 teaspoon extract (almond, chocolate, hazelnut, vanilla)

½ to 2 teaspoons fresh citrus juice

½ to 2 teaspoons grated citrus zest

2 tablespoons cocoa/cacao powder

1 tablespoon ground coffee

1 to 3 teaspoons pumpkin pie spice

½ to 1 teaspoon ground ginger (or 1 to 2 teaspoons peeled, minced fresh ginger)

Moisture ---------- *and* ----------> Sticky Sweet

½ CUP TOTAL
Choose one
or combine

Applesauce

Banana, mashed

Pumpkin purée

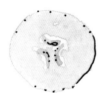

3 TABLESPOONS TOTAL
Choose one
or combine

Blackstrap molasses

Brown rice syrup

Raw, unpasteurized honey

Maple syrup

Texture

½ CUP TOTAL
Choose one

Dried coconut (shredded or flakes), toasted or raw

Dried fruit (pome, berries, tropical, stone)

3 Fold in Special Additions (if using) until incorporated. Use an ice cream scoop or spoon to place 2-inch (5 cm) dollops of dough on a parchment-lined baking sheet. Press flat or keep in macaroon shape—the shape won't change as it bakes. Bake for 25 to 30 minutes, until the edges brown.

Remove from the oven; cool on the baking sheet. Store in a container in the fridge for two weeks.

Special Additions

Choose as many as you like, or skip altogether

1 to 2 teaspoons tea leaves, ground in coffee/spice grinder (chai, Earl Grey, rooibos, etc.)

½ cup (90 g) chocolate (dark or white; chopped or chips)

¼ to ½ cup (40 to 80 g) crystallized ginger, chopped

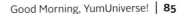

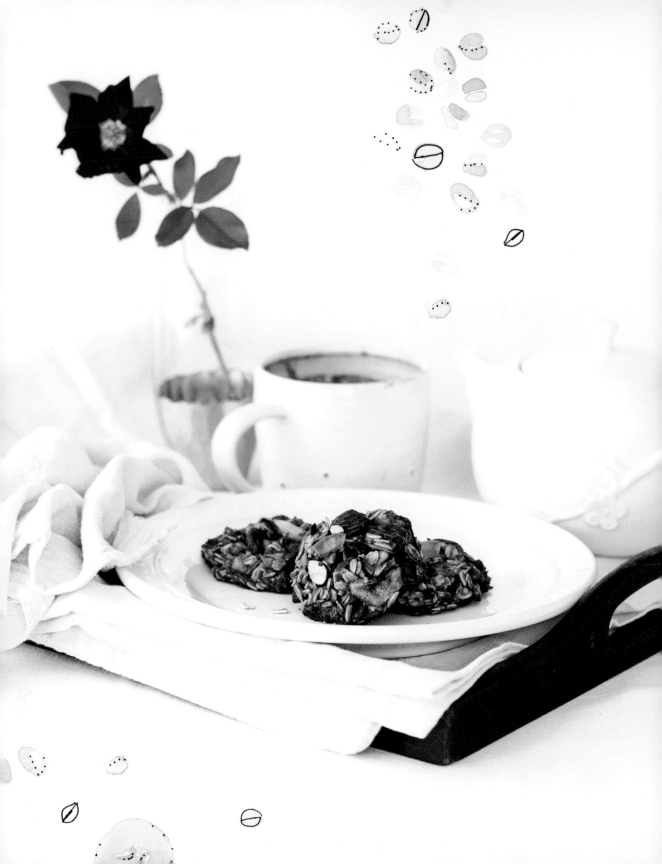

Banana Chocolate Chip Breakfast Cookies

The comfort of banana bread and a bowl of warm oatmeal with extra texture from toasted coconut and dark chocolate chunks— always a winning combination.

MAKES 12 TO 14

½ cup (70 g) raw, unsalted almonds, chopped into tiny pieces

½ cup (40 g) flaked or shredded dried coconut

1 cup (80 g) rolled oats

½ teaspoon ground cinnamon

½ teaspoon ground psyllium husk

½ teaspoon sea salt

3 tablespoons maple syrup

½ cup (110 g) mashed banana

¼ cup (60 ml) dairy-free milk or water, gently warmed

2 tablespoons unrefined coconut oil, gently warmed to liquid

2 teaspoons fresh lemon juice

1 teaspoon vanilla extract

½ cup (90 g) chopped dairy-free dark chocolate (about one 3-ounce/85 g bar)

1. Preheat the oven to 350°F (180°C). Line a baking sheet with unbleached parchment paper and spread the chopped almonds in one layer on the sheet so they have room to roast mostly untouched on all sides. Pop in the oven for 7 minutes. Transfer the nuts to a large mixing bowl and scatter the coconut on the sheet; roast for 3 to 4 minutes, until starting to brown, and add to the bowl with the nuts. Set the lined baking sheet aside.

2. Add the oats, cinnamon, psyllium, and salt to the mixing bowl and stir until well mixed. In a small bowl, stir together the mashed banana, warm dairy-free milk, warm coconut oil, lemon juice, and vanilla extract until well mixed. Fold together the wet and dry ingredients, and then fold in the chopped chocolate until thoroughly incorporated.

3. Use an ice cream scoop or spoon to place 2-inch (5 cm) dollops of dough on the lined baking sheet. Press flat if you like or keep in macaroon shape—the shape won't change as it bakes. Bake for 25 to 30 minutes, until the edges start to brown. Remove from the oven; cool completely on the baking sheet. Store in the fridge in an airtight glass container for up to two weeks.

Pumpkin-Pecan Breakfast Cookies

The flavors in these breakfast cookies continue to evolve after the first bite through to the last. It's a flavorful combination of spicy ginger and warming cloves, cinnamon, and nutmeg with pops of sweet from juicy raisins—the flavors of fall.

MAKES 12 TO 14

½ cup (50 g) raw, unsalted pecans, chopped into tiny pieces

1 cup (80 g) rolled oats

2 tablespoons Sucanat

1 tablespoon pumpkin pie spice

½ teaspoon ground psyllium husk

½ teaspoon sea salt

½ cup (120 ml) dairy-free milk or water, gently warmed

½ cup (120 g) pumpkin purée

3 tablespoons maple syrup

2 tablespoons unrefined coconut oil, gently warmed to liquid

2 teaspoons fresh lemon juice

1 teaspoon peeled, grated fresh ginger—almost a pulp

1 teaspoon vanilla extract

½ cup (75 g) raisins

½ cup (80 g) crystallized ginger, chopped into tiny pieces (optional)

1. Preheat the oven to 350°F (180°C). Line a baking sheet with unbleached parchment paper and spread the chopped pecans in one layer on the sheet so they have room to roast mostly untouched on all sides. Pop in the oven to roast for 7 minutes. Transfer the nuts to a mixing bowl and set the lined baking sheet aside.

2. Add the oats, Sucanat, pumpkin pie spice, psyllium, and salt to the mixing bowl and stir until well mixed. In a small bowl, stir together the warm dairy-free milk, pumpkin purée, maple syrup, warm coconut oil, lemon juice, fresh ginger, and vanilla extract until well mixed. Fold together the wet and dry ingredients, and then fold in the raisins and crystallized ginger until thoroughly incorporated.

3. Use an ice cream scoop or spoon to place 2-inch (5 cm) dollops of dough on the parchment-lined baking sheet. Press flat if you like or keep in macaroon shape—the shape won't change as it bakes. Bake for 25 to 30 minutes, until the edges start to brown. Remove from the oven; cool completely on the baking sheet. Store in the fridge in an airtight glass container for up to two weeks.

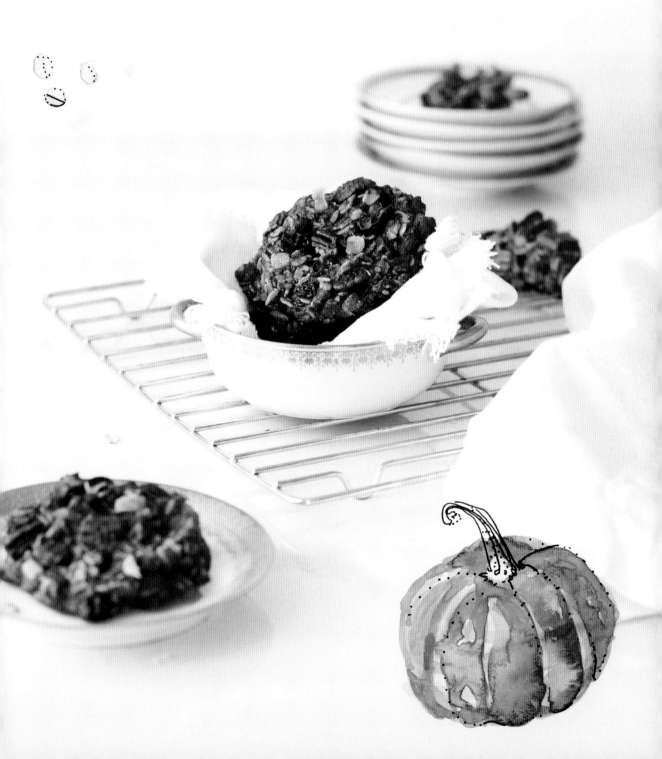

Compotes & Fruit Butters

Compotes and fruit butters are easy to make and a
great way to use up almost-over-the-hill fruit.
Fruit butter is often prepared in a slow cooker for up
to 5 hours—do that if you like—but this template
is for "quick" fruit butter.

Into canning? Use your know-how to store creations
for months. Otherwise, store in a jar in the fridge
for a few weeks, or freeze for a few months, and eat up
as you see fit. Compotes and fruit butters take
French toast, Pancakes & Waffles (page 55), Warm Cereals
(page 73), Nice Cream (page 279), Parfaits (page 99),
and Coconut Yogurt (page 94) to the next level.

For fun, add 1 tablespoon of brandy, cognac,
Chambord, or Cointreau or ¼ cup (60 ml)
wine or hard cider.

Compote combo on this page: Rosewater & plum.

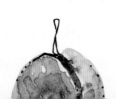

What you need no matter what:

Pinch or two sea salt

¼ cup (60 ml) or more water to reach desired thickness

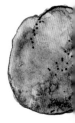

1 Place Fruit, Acid, Sweet (if using), **salt** to taste, Flavor (if using), and the **water** in a large pot and bring to a boil over medium heat. Reduce the heat and continue cooking over medium-low heat for 10 to 20 minutes, until thickened and the fruit is broken down. At this point, the compote is done. Remove from the heat and cool. For fruit butter: Purée the compote until smooth. For thicker fruit butter, return to the pot and simmer to desired thickness or jump to Step 2, but note: The mixture thickens as it cools.

Fruit ----- *and* -----→ Acid ----- *and/or* -----→ Sweet

3 CUPS (FRESH OR FROZEN) WASHED, PITTED/CORED, EVENLY CHOPPED TOTAL
Choose one or combine

Pome fruit (any kind)

Stone fruit (any kind)

Berries (any kind)

Tomatoes (any kind), blanched and peeled

Pineapple, peeled

Mango, peeled

Pumpkin, peeled

Melon, peeled and seeded

1 TO 2 TEASPOONS TOTAL
Choose one or combine

Apple cider vinegar

Citrus juice

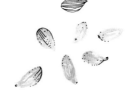

1 TO 4 TABLESPOONS TOTAL
Choose one or combine or skip altogether

Raw, unpasteurized honey

Maple syrup

Sucanat

Coconut sugar

Flavor

Choose as many as you like, or skip altogether

½ to 2 teaspoons grated citrus zest

1 to 2 teaspoons balsamic vinegar

1 to 3 teaspoons chopped fresh herbs (mint, thyme, basil, cilantro)

1 teaspoon fennel seeds

¼ to 1 teaspoon fresh-cracked pink peppercorn

Pinch to ¼ teaspoon cayenne pepper

Seeds from 1 vanilla bean pod

½ to 1 teaspoon ground ginger (or 1 to 3 teaspoons peeled, minced fresh ginger)

¼ to 1 teaspoon extract (vanilla, almond)

¼ teaspoon orange blossom or rosewater

Pinch to ¼ teaspoon ground cardamom

¼ to 1 teaspoon ground cinnamon

Pinch to ¼ teaspoon ground cloves

Pinch to ¼ teaspoon ground nutmeg

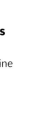

2 After the compote has cooled a bit, to make it thicker or to add texture, stir in Thickener over medium heat for 2 to 3 minutes, then cool. Transfer to glass jars and refrigerate until ready to enjoy. Compote and fruit butters keep for weeks in a glass container in the fridge, and months in the freezer.

Thickener

Choose one or skip altogether

½ to 2 teaspoons chia seeds

Slurry: 1 teaspoon arrowroot starch/flour dissolved in 2 tablespoons water

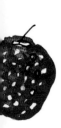
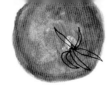

Strawberry-Tomato & Basil Compote

A surprising combination that's delicious piled on vanilla bean Nice Cream (page 279) and layered in a sour homemade Coconut Yogurt (page 94).

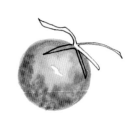

SERVES 8+

2½ cups (415 g) quartered strawberries

½ cup (90 g) blanched, peeled, diced tomato (about 1 small)

¼ cup (60 ml) raw, unpasteurized honey

¼ cup (60 ml) water

1 tablespoon finely chopped fresh basil

1 teaspoon fresh lime juice

Pinch or two sea salt

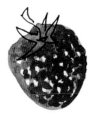

1. Place the strawberries, tomato, honey, water, basil, lime juice, and salt to taste in a large pot and bring to a boil over medium heat. Reduce the heat and continue cooking over low heat for 10 to 20 minutes, until thickened and the fruit is broken down—help it along by mashing with a wooden spoon.

2. Remove from the heat and cool—the mixture will thicken. Transfer to glass jars and chill in the fridge until ready to use. The compote keeps for weeks in an airtight glass container in the fridge, and months in the freezer.

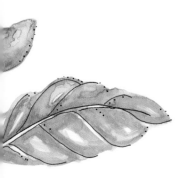

Spiced Pear Butter

In the fall, I go bananas at the orchards and farmers' markets for apples and pears. This is a great way to use up all the goods. Use this butter to add flavor to Warm Cereals (page 73), spread it on toast with coconut oil, or use it to fill Hand Pies (page 243).

SERVES 8+

1 vanilla bean pod

3 cups (480 g) cored, chopped pear (any kind, skin on or off—chef's choice)

½ cup (60 ml) water

3 tablespoons maple syrup

2 teaspoons peeled, grated fresh ginger—almost a pulp

1½ teaspoons ground cinnamon

1 teaspoon apple cider vinegar

¼ teaspoon ground nutmeg

Pinch or two sea salt

Pinch of ground cardamom

Pinch of ground cloves

1. Lightly press your vanilla bean pod so it lies flat on a cutting board. Carefully slice all the way down its length with a sharp knife and open. Use the back of your knife or the back of a spoon to scrape out the caviar-like seeds and toss into a large pot. Add the pears, water, maple syrup, ginger, cinnamon, vinegar, nutmeg, salt to taste, cardamom, and cloves to the pot with the vanilla and bring to a boil over medium heat.

2. Reduce the heat and continue cooking over medium-low heat for 10 to 20 minutes, until thickened and fruit is broken down—you can help it along by mashing with a wooden spoon. Remove from the heat.

3. Use an immersion blender, standing blender, or food processor to purée the compote until smooth. If you want the butter to be thicker, return it to the pot and continue to cook on a low simmer until the desired thickness is achieved. Fruit Butter keeps for weeks in an airtight glass container in the fridge, and months in the freezer.

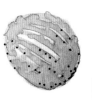

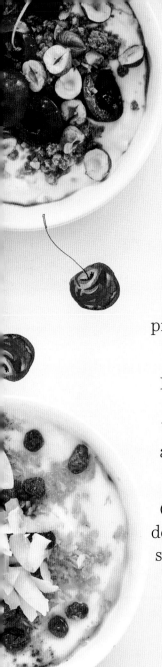

Coconut Yogurt

Most store-bought yogurt is full of sugar, preservatives, dyes, and thickeners, and they're also pasteurized, which kills any probiotic benefit.

Dairy-free cultured yogurt is a twist on traditional practices that are thousands of years old. You're creating a feast for beneficial bacteria, and as they munch, they ferment and sour—the result is delicious, gut-friendly yogurt.

Opening young coconuts can be a challenge if you don't have special tools like a cleaver or a Coco Jack, so you can make a little coconut meat go a long way by stretching the mix with canned coconut milk.

For best results, use raw, organic ingredients, and note: The warmer the kitchen, the faster the fermentation.

Yogurt bowl combos on this spread clockwise from top left: Hazelnut granola & cherry; almond & chamomile-apple compote; blueberry, pecan, chia & lemon zest; mixed berry compote, crystallized ginger, pepitas & walnuts; cinnamon, nutmeg, carrots, maple syrup, raisins & toasted coconut.

Learn more about the benefits, safety, and possibilities of fermented foods: yumuniverse.com/?s=fermented

3+ CUPS (675 G)
PREP TIME: 5 TO 15 MINUTES
FERMENTATION TIME: 3 TO 7 DAYS

What you need no matter what:

1 cup (80 g) young coconut meat

1 refrigerated probiotic capsule (any kind you like)

1 Place the **coconut meat,** Cream, and Liquid (start with less, add more as you go) in the blender and mix until ultra-smooth. Add more liquid if needed until you reach a melted ice cream consistency. The yogurt will thicken, losing 10 to 15 percent water as it ferments over the next few days.

Cream ---- *and* ---> Liquid

1 CUP (240 ML OR 80 G) TOTAL
Choose one or combine

Canned coconut
milk (full fat, not
reduced fat)

Young coconut meat

¾ TO 1½ CUPS
(180 TO 300 ML)
TOTAL
Choose one

Pure water

Raw coconut water

Unpasteurized, raw,
dairy-free milk

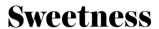

How to open a young coconut: yumuniverse.com/how-to-open-a-young-coconut

2 Transfer the mixture to a clean glass bowl using a wooden or silicone spoon—the bacteria don't like metal. Open the **probiotic capsule** and sprinkle the contents into the yogurt and stir. Cover with a cloth napkin and secure with a rubber band. Place in a warm spot in the kitchen out of sunlight for 1 to 5 days. Use a clean nonmetal utensil to sample after 1 day—let it ferment longer until the desired sourness is achieved. Every day will yield more sourness.

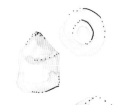

3 Once the desired sourness is achieved, swirl in Sweetness, if you like. Store the yogurt in an airtight glass container in the fridge for 2 to 4 weeks. Yogurt will continue to ferment and sour, just at a slower pace.

Sweetness

1 TABLESPOON TO ¼ CUP TOTAL
Choose as many as you like,
or skip altogether

Raw, unpasteurized
honey

Maple syrup

Sucanat

Blended fruit or
Compote (page 90)

Savory Chickpea & Fresh Mint Yogurt Bowl

This recipe has all the tasty flavors of homemade falafel—deconstructed. If you want to use homemade Yogurt (page 94), you'll need to prepare it 1 to 3 days in advance. So, make a big batch and enjoy it with all the recipes that call for yogurt in this book.

SERVES 2+

1 cup (225 g) unsweetened Coconut Yogurt (make 1 to 3 days in advance from page 94, or use store-bought dairy-free yogurt)

½ cup (65 g) diced cucumber

¼ cup (5 g) loosely packed fresh mint leaves, chopped

1 to 2 teaspoons unrefined coconut oil or grapeseed oil

2 cups (330 g) cooked chickpeas (roughly ¾ cup/160 g dry; see page 11)

1 shallot, minced

3 to 4 leaves kale, stems removed and chopped (any kind)

2 tablespoons chopped fresh parsley

1 teaspoon ground coriander

1 teaspoon ground cumin

½ teaspoon sea salt, plus more to taste

¼ teaspoon ground cinnamon

Pinch cayenne pepper

Pinch ground cardamom

1 to 2 cloves garlic, minced

Fresh-ground black pepper

1 lemon

1 to 2 small radishes, sliced

1 Make a fresh Mint Yogurt by combining the yogurt, cucumber, and mint in a small bowl. Pop in the fridge to chill.

2 In a skillet heated to medium, add the oil and sauté the chickpeas and shallot for 5 minutes, or until the shallot softens. Add the kale, parsley, coriander, cumin, salt, cinnamon, cayenne, and cardamom; cook together for 5 more minutes. Add the garlic and stir together for 3 minutes. Season with black pepper and more salt if you like, and don't forget a generous squeeze of fresh lemon juice to taste. Serve topped with the radish and chilled Mint Yogurt and enjoy.

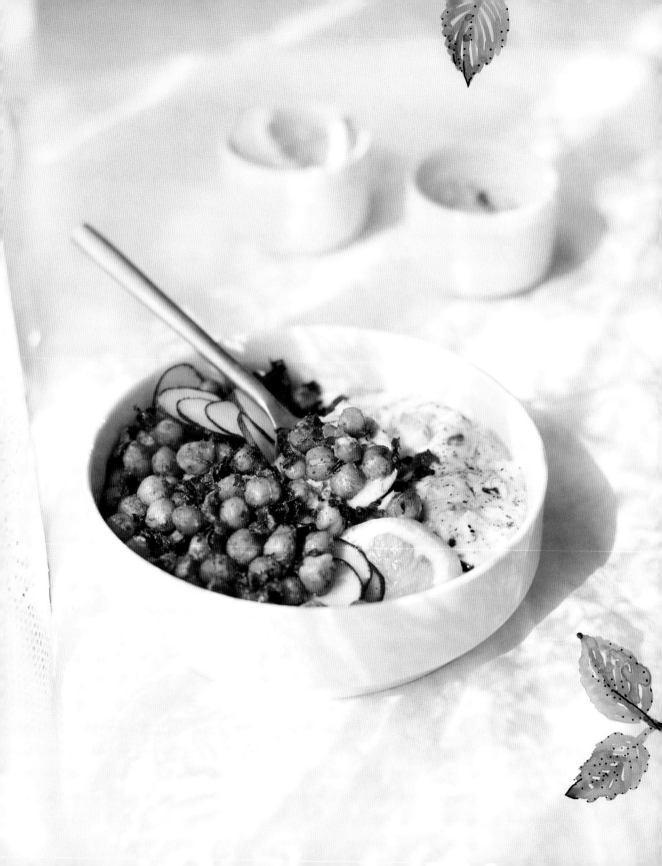

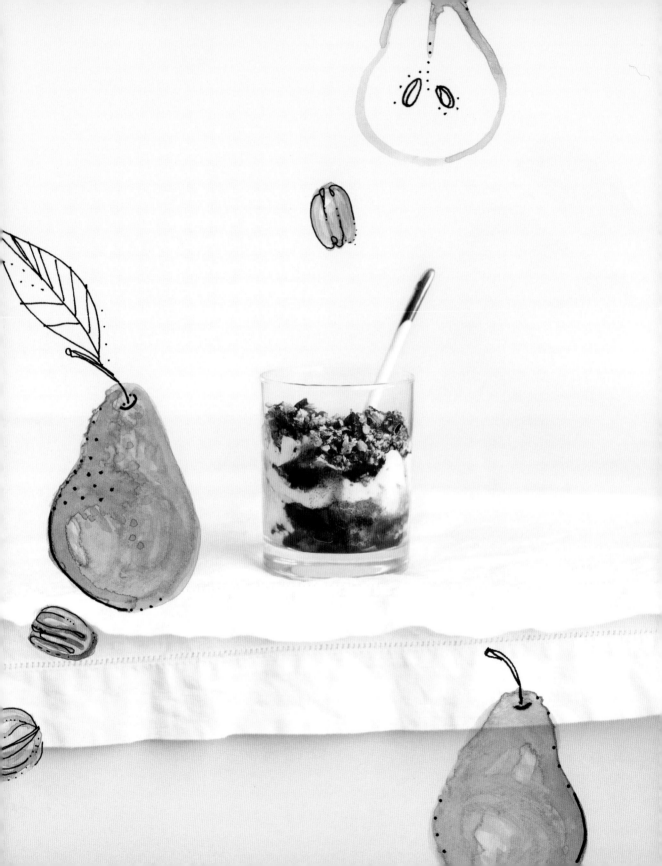

Maple-Spiced Pear & Toasted Pecan Parfait

It's breakfast, it's a snack, it's dessert, it's also easy to throw
together on the fly or the night before you want it.
You'll just need to make a batch of Coconut Yogurt (page 94)
1 to 3 days in advance, or use your favorite store-bought variety.

SERVES 4+

Maple-Spiced Pear Compote

2 not-too-ripe pears, peeled, cored, and chopped

¼ cup (60 ml) maple syrup

1½ teaspoons apple cider vinegar

1 teaspoon ground cinnamon

¾ teaspoon peeled, grated fresh ginger—almost a pulp

½ teaspoon vanilla extract (or seeds from ½ vanilla bean pod)

¼ teaspoon ground cardamom

A few pinches sea salt

—

2 cups (200 g) raw, unsalted pecans

2 cups (450 g) Coconut Yogurt (make 1 to 3 days in advance from page 94, or use store-bought dairy-free yogurt)

1 teaspoon chia seeds

1. Combine the pears, maple syrup, vinegar, cinnamon, ginger, vanilla, cardamom, and a pinch of salt in a large pot and bring to a boil over medium-high heat. Reduce to a simmer and cook until the fruit is a jam-like consistency, 10 to 15 minutes. Remove from the heat and cool until ready to use—the mixture will thicken as it cools.

2. Preheat the oven to 350°F (180°C) and line a baking sheet with unbleached parchment paper. Spread the pecans on the sheet in one layer so they have room to roast mostly untouched on all sides. Sprinkle with a pinch of salt and pop in the oven for 7 minutes. Remove, chop, and set aside.

3. Create an assembly line. Set out four 4-inch (10 cm) tall vessels that you'd like to layer your parfaits in and bring the compote, yogurt, chia seeds, and pecans within reach.

4. Spoon some compote into the bottom of each vessel, then top with a layer of chopped pecans and a sprinkling of chia seeds. Add some yogurt to each. Repeat until full. Chill and serve, or enjoy immediately.

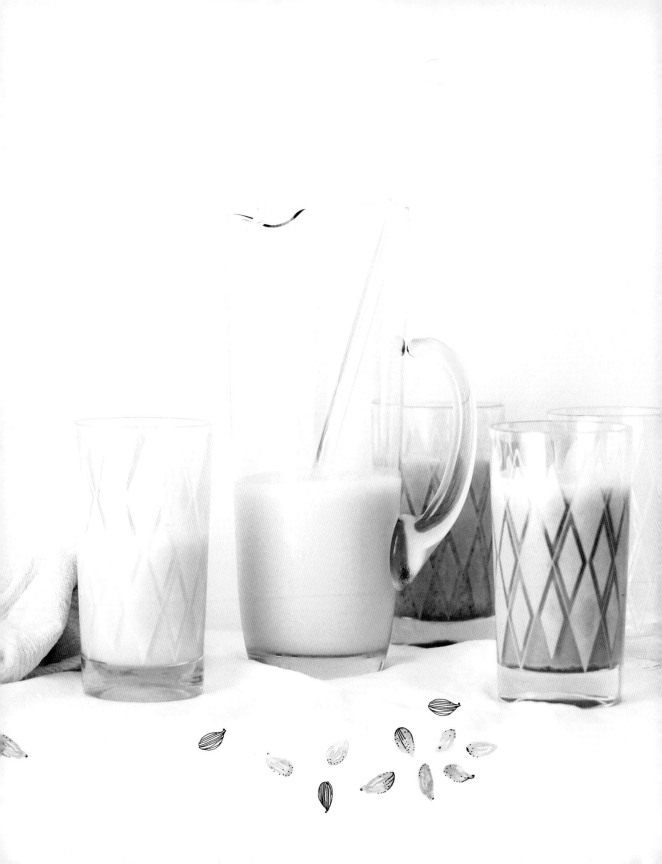

Dairy-Free Milks

Making dairy-free milk at home is easy, tastes better than store-bought, and has the right amount of preservatives and suspicious additives: ahem, zero.

If you're in a hurry, use nut or seed butter as your base. Or soak nuts and seeds while you sleep for decadent, easy, nutrient-rich milk in the morning. Add cacao, berries, or fragrant spices like cardamom, cinnamon, even cayenne for some kick. And toasted coconut, seeds, and grains for nutty, rich flavor before blending.

Dairy-Free Milk combos on this spread left to right:
Coconut-cardamom; honey & cashew; poppy seed;
strawberry-almond; coconut-hemp.

Dairy-Free Milks

8+ SERVINGS
PREP TIME: 15 TO 35 MINUTES

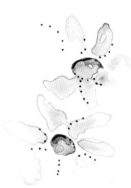

All you need is a blender and, to strain, a tight-weave cheesecloth, scrap of muslin, nut milk bag, or piece of a recycled curtain sheer.

Psst: Fold leftover pulp into a cracker recipe based off of page 112.

What you need no matter what:

Pinch or two sea salt

1   If using nuts and/or large seeds for your Base, soak, drain, and rinse well. Or roast in an oven heated to 350°F (180°C) for 5 to 7 minutes until brown and smelling nutty and divine. Transfer to the blender.

Base

Choose one or combine

Choose any in combination totaling 1 cup; nuts, seeds, and grains are raw, unsalted... **AND/OR**   - - - - - - - ->   *Choose any in combination totaling 3 tablespoons*

Almonds	Hazelnuts	Pine nuts
Amaranth	Hemp seeds	Poppy seeds
Brazil nuts	Macadamia nuts	Quinoa
Brown rice	Millet	Sesame seeds
Buckwheat groats	Oats	Sunflower seeds
Cashews	Pecans	Walnuts
Coconut (dry flaked/ or shredded, or raw)	Pepitas/pumpkin seeds	

Nut butter, unsalted

Seed butter, unsalted

2 Add Liquid, Flavor, Sweetness (if using), and the **salt** to taste to the blender; blend until ultra-smooth, about 1 minute. Strain and squeeze the mixture through a cheesecloth if needed.

Liquid ---- *and* ----> Flavor

4 CUPS (960 ML) TOTAL
Choose one or combine

Pure water

Coconut water

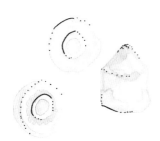

Choose one or combine, or skip altogether

2 to 4 tablespoons cacao nibs

¼ teaspoon ground cardamom

¼ teaspoon cayenne pepper

1 to 2 teaspoons ground cinnamon

¼ teaspoon ground cloves

¼ teaspoon ground nutmeg

1 teaspoon extract (almond, chocolate, hazelnut, vanilla)

Seeds from 1 vanilla bean pod

1 to 2 tablespoons grated orange zest

2 tablespoons ground coffee

⅛ teaspoon orange blossom or rosewater

1 to 4 teaspoons fresh herbs (thyme, lavender, rosemary, mint)

½ to 1 teaspoon ground ginger (or 1 to 2 teaspoons peeled, minced fresh ginger)

1 to 2 tablespoons tea leaves (chai, chicory root, Earl Grey, green, licorice root, rooibos)

Sweetness Choose one or combine, or skip altogether

1 to 4 tablespoons brown rice syrup

1 to 3 tablespoons coconut sugar

1 to 4 tablespoons raw, unpasteurized honey

1 to 4 tablespoons maple syrup

1 to 4 tablespoons blackstrap molasses

1 to 3 tablespoons Sucanat

1 to 3 tablespoons rapadura

3 to 5 dates (any kind), pitted

---

3 Transfer the milk back to the blender if adding Boost, and blend until smooth. Enjoy or chill in fridge. Milk may separate—this is normal—just give it a shake or a blend before serving.

Boost Choose one or combine, or skip altogether

1 teaspoon sunflower lecithin (adds thickness)

1 to 4 teaspoons maca powder

1 to 4 teaspoons chia seeds

1 to 2 teaspoons spirulina

1 teaspoon ground turmeric

1 to 4 teaspoons bee pollen

1 to 2 tablespoons cocoa/cacao powder

1 to 4 teaspoons greens powder (any kind)

1 to 2 teaspoons matcha

1 to 4 tablespoons plant protein powder

¼ cup (35 g) fresh or frozen fruit (pome, tropical, stone, berries)

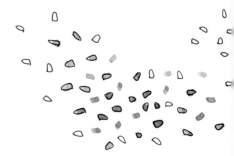

Toasted Black Sesame Seed Milk

This milk is great for anyone looking for a dairy-free milk that's nut-free and full of rich flavor. You can make this milk using golden sesames if you like—you won't get the unusual color, but you will get the unique taste. You can skip the sweetener for this recipe if you like, too. Make it your own.

SERVES 2+

1 cup (145 g) raw, unsalted black sesame seeds

4 cups (960 ml) water

3 tablespoons raw, unpasteurized honey, or more to taste

⅛ teaspoon ground cardamom (optional)

Pinch sea salt

1   Preheat the oven to 350°F (180°C) and line a baking sheet with parchment paper. Scatter the sesame seeds on the sheet and toast for 7 to 10 minutes, until smelling nutty. Toss into the blender.

2   Add the water, honey, cardamom (if using), and salt and blend until ultra-smooth, about 1 minute. Strain and squeeze the mixture through a cheesecloth or nut milk bag. Feel free to add more honey. Enjoy right away or chill in the fridge. Give it a shake before serving.

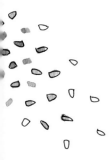

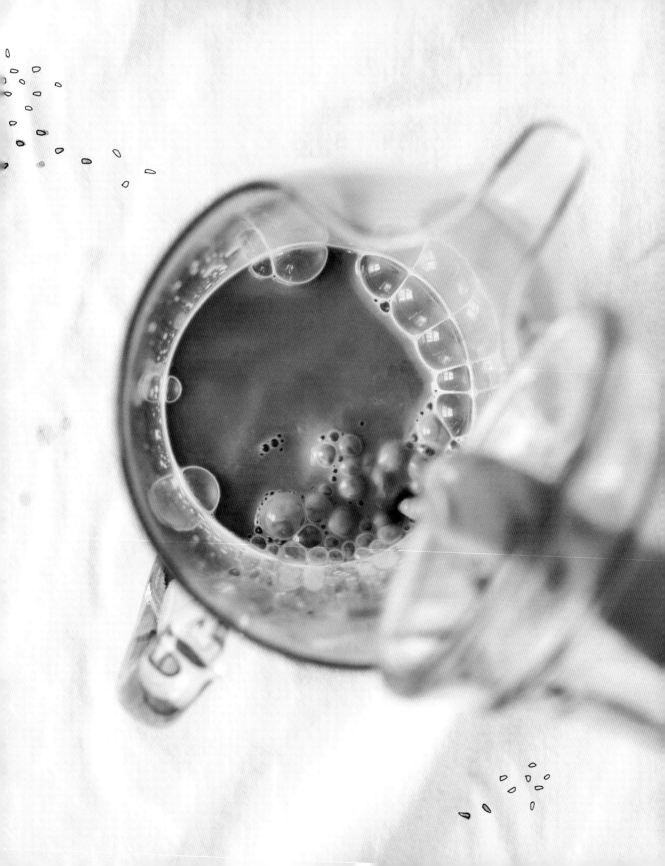

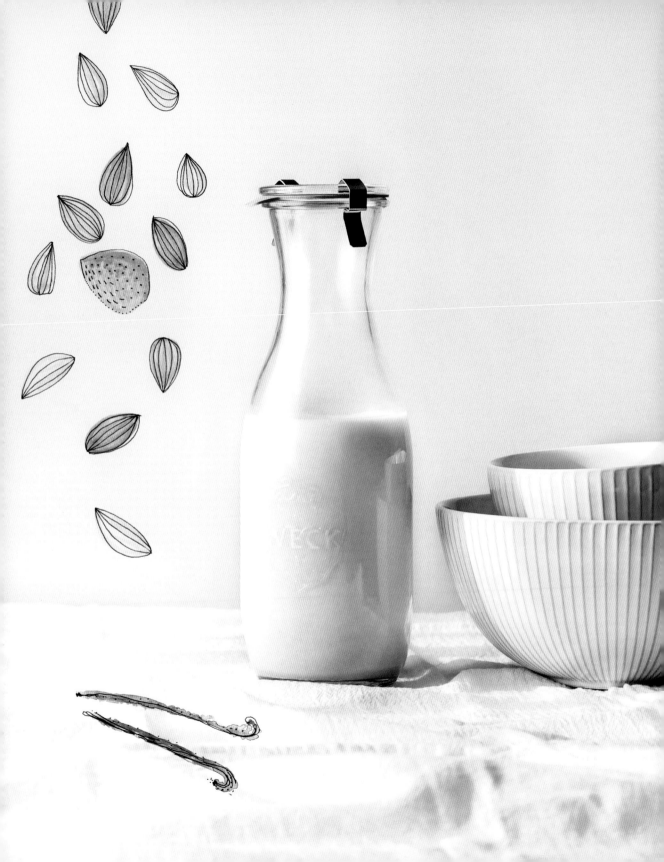

Vanilla-Almond Milk

A staple for warm cereals, smoothies, and granola, this recipe combines rich, creamy almonds and fragrant vanilla bean. For a special treat, blend in fresh berries and maybe a drop or two of rosewater or orange blossom water.

Want a simple, everyday version of this classic dairy-free milk? Blend almond butter with vanilla extract, dates, a pinch of sea salt and water; skip the straining. The dates will make a froth that is heaven spooned onto a chai tea!

SERVES 2+

1 cup (145 g) raw, unsalted almonds

1 vanilla bean pod

4 cups (960 ml) coconut water

2 Medjool dates, pitted

⅛ teaspoon rosewater (optional)

Pinch sea salt

1. Place the almonds in a bowl of water and soak for 8 to 12 hours (while you sleep is a good time). Drain, rinse, and transfer to the blender. Press the vanilla pod flat and slice through the top layer lengthwise; open the pod and use the back of a knife to scrape out the gorgeous seeds inside. Tap the seeds into the blender.

2. Add the coconut water, dates, rosewater (if using), and salt and blend until ultra-smooth, about 1 minute. Strain and squeeze the mixture through a cheesecloth. Enjoy right away or chill the in fridge. Give it a shake before serving with cereal, granola, tea, or coffee.

Decadent Pecan Milk Hot Cocoa
(with all the fixings)

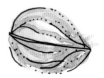

Any dairy-free milk creations can be served warm—
it makes them even more comforting, like this
decadent hot cocoa. I have a few optional ingredients listed
here to make this recipe unforgettable, but push it
even further if you like with a pinch of cayenne and
some ground cinnamon—a hot cocoa to rival them all!

SERVES 4

1 cup (100 g) raw, unsalted pecans

4 cups (960 ml) water

5 Medjool dates, pitted

3 tablespoons maple syrup

2 tablespoons cocoa/cacao powder

1 teaspoon vanilla extract

Pinch sea salt

One 13.5-ounce (400 ml) can coconut milk, chilled (optional)

¼ cup (40 g) shaved/grated chocolate bar (optional)

¼ cup (60 ml) Butterscotch (optional, page 33)

1   Place the pecans in a bowl of water and soak for 8 to 12 hours (while you sleep is a good time). Drain, rinse, and transfer to the blender.

2   Add the water and blend until ultra-smooth, 1 to 2 minutes. Strain the mixture through a cheesecloth and transfer the milk back to the rinsed blender. Add the dates, maple syrup, cacao, vanilla extract, and salt; blend until smooth and transfer to a large pot heated to medium. Bring to a boil. Remove from the heat and pour into mugs.

3   If you like, spoon some cream from the top of the can of coconut milk onto the cocoa and top with shaved chocolate and a drizzle or three of Butterscotch. Yes!

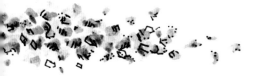

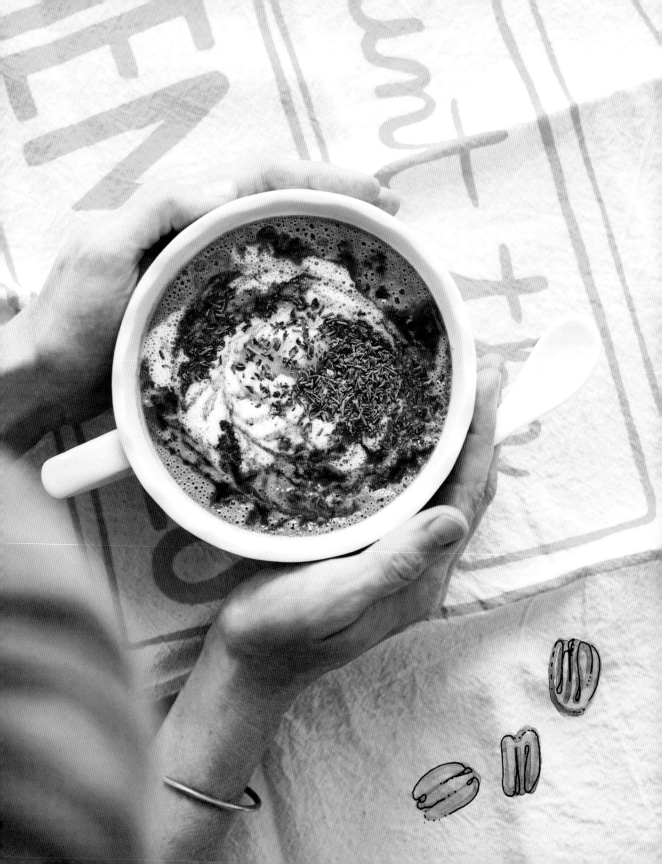

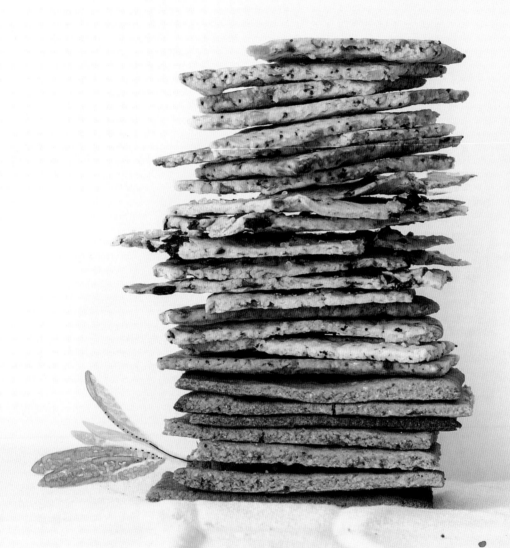

Cracker combos shown here top to bottom:
Dulse & black pepper; Sun-Dried Tomato &
Herb (page 114); cinnamon & honey.

Munch & Lunch

WHEN YOU THINK OF SNACKING, you likely have visions of crackers, fries, dips, and tasty salted, crunchy things, right? But when many folks hear "gluten-free" and "dairy-free," they assume that these comforts are now out of the question. I know I used to.

I didn't want to give up on the foods that feel like they're in my DNA, and I can bet you don't, either. This is why I created alternatives I could feel great about.

The following pages illustrate that snacky staples like cream cheese, fun eats like tots, and outside-the-comfort-zone goodness like easy (yes, easy) fermented veggies add more flavor and "life" to our life—we just have to dial up the plant factor. So, turn this page to discover crave-worthy on-the-go snacks, side dishes, appetizers, and ideas for lunch itself!

Crackers

12+ SERVINGS
BAKE TIME: 10 TO 15 MINUTES

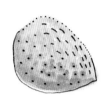

It's hard to find tasty gluten-free crackers on store shelves that aren't void of nutrients or loaded with starches. Well, let me tell you, it's easy and fun to bake some at home in as little as 15 minutes.

These crackers can be made 100 percent with almond flour or mixed with another flour. Almond flour adds buttery richness and extra protein to the dough—use blanched for the best flavor and texture. I often double or triple the batch and store in the fridge for when I want something crunchy. They last for weeks in an airtight glass container. Crumble them into Epic Salads (page 195), serve them with Dips & Spreads (page 137), plunge them into Soups (page 175), and load them up with veggies, greens, and spreads for mini cracker sandwiches.

What you need no matter what:

½ cup (55 g) blanched almond flour

¼ teaspoon baking powder

¼ teaspoon sea salt, or more to taste

1 tablespoon chilled unrefined coconut oil

2 tablespoons cold water, plus more if needed

1 Preheat the oven to 375°F (190°C). In a bowl using a fork, or in a food processor fitted with the S-blade, mix Flour with the **almond flour, baking powder,** and **salt.** Cut the **oil** in until uniformly crumbly.

Flour

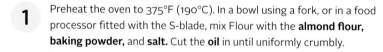

½ CUP TOTAL
Choose one
or combine

Blanched
almond flour

Brown rice flour

Oat flour

Sorghum flour

Teff flour

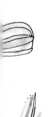

2 Evenly incorporate Flavor (if using), 1 tablespoon of the **cold water,** and Fold-Ins (if using). Use your hands to form a ball of dough. Too dry? Add 1 teaspoon water at a time until the dough forms a ball, but note: Less is more.

Flavor

Optional

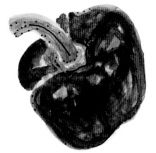

Choose any of these in combination **OR** -> *Choose one of these by itself*

1 teaspoon extract (almond, vanilla)

½ to 1 teaspoon grated citrus zest

1 to 4 teaspoons chopped fresh herbs

1 to 2 tablespoons spice/seasoning mix (ranch, taco, curry, jerk, herbes de Provence, Italian, za'atar spice blend)

1 tablespoon caraway seeds

1 tablespoon Sucanat or coconut sugar

¼ to 1 teaspoon fresh-cracked black pepper

¼ to 1 teaspoon ground cinnamon

1 teaspoon raw, unpasteurized honey or blackstrap molasses

1 to 4 teaspoons cocoa/cacao powder

1 tablespoon dulse flakes

½ to 1 teaspoon nutritional yeast

Fold-Ins

1 TO 4 TABLESPOONS TOTAL
Choose one or combine, or skip altogether; mince into tiny pieces

Sun-dried tomato

Nuts & seeds (raw or toasted)

Onion or shallot (raw or sautéed)

Dried fruit

Garlic, minced

Red bell pepper, seeded, ribs removed (raw or roasted)

3 Place the dough ball on a baking-sheet-sized piece of parchment paper and lay another sheet on top. Use a rolling pin to flatten to ⅛ inch (3 mm) between the sheets. Peel back the top sheet and sculpt the dough into a rectangle, then score cracker shapes—punch holes with a fork if you like. Slide the dough and parchment onto a baking sheet. Bake for 10 to 15 minutes, until the edges begin to brown. Remove from the oven; cool on the sheet.

Sun-Dried Tomato & Herb Crackers

These crackers have a bit of a pizza vibe—cheesy and herby, with flavorful pops of sun-dried tomato. They're delicious solo and spread with hummus. This recipe plays with some textural finishing salt, but you can easily skip it and use ¼ teaspoon fine-ground sea salt in the dough only.

MAKES 12+

½ cup (55 g) blanched almond flour

½ cup (60 g) sorghum flour

¼ teaspoon baking powder

Pinch sea salt

Maldon or other finishing salt

1 tablespoon chilled unrefined coconut oil

2 garlic cloves, minced

2 teaspoons chopped fresh basil

2 teaspoons chopped fresh oregano

1 teaspoon nutritional yeast

2 tablespoons cold water, plus more if needed

3 tablespoons minced sun-dried tomatoes

1 Preheat the oven to 375°F (190°C). Cut two baking-sheet-sized pieces of unbleached parchment paper; set aside.

2 In a bowl using a fork, or in a food processor fitted with the S-blade, mix together the almond flour, sorghum flour, baking powder, and salt. Cut the oil into the flour mixture until uniformly crumbly. Stir in the garlic, basil, oregano, and nutritional yeast, and add 2 tablespoons of the cold water until crumbles start to stick together. Incorporate the sun-dried tomatoes and use your hands to try to form a ball of dough. If it's too dry, add 1 teaspoon water at a time until the dough forms a ball, but note: Less is more; work the dough well with your hands first.

3 Place the dough ball on one piece of parchment paper and lay the other sheet on top. Use a rolling pin to flatten to ⅛ inch (3 mm) between the sheets. Peel back the top sheet and use a knife to sculpt the dough into a rectangle, or leave the edges rustic—baker's choice—then score cracker shapes. Sprinkle with finishing salt. Slide the dough and parchment onto a baking sheet. Bake for 10 to 15 minutes, until the edges begin to brown. Remove from the oven and cool on the baking sheet.

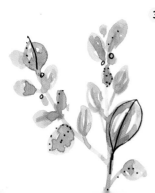

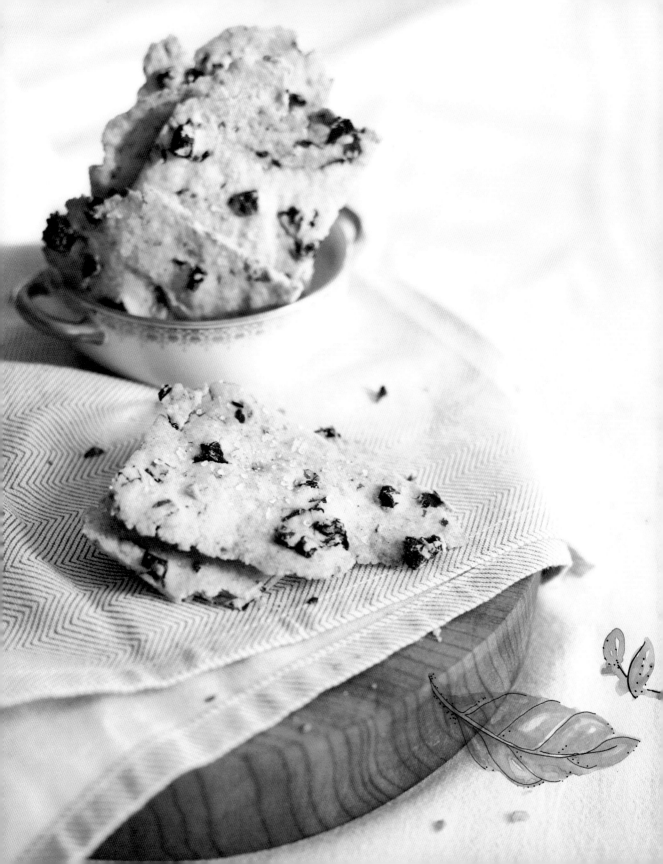

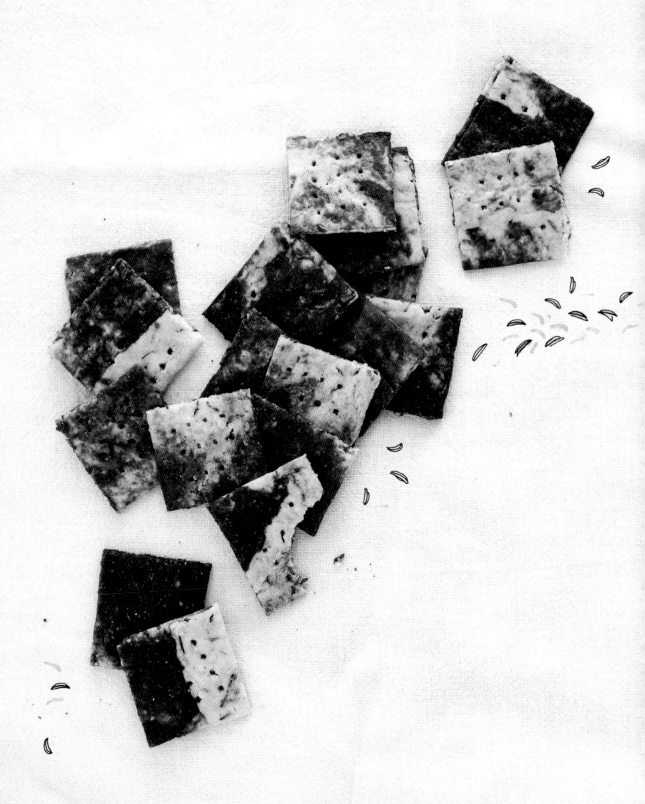

Caraway Swirl Crackers

I'm pushing the basic template techniques a bit here—combining different colored doughs to make some extra pretty crackers. These are inspired by a classic rye swirl bread my father used to have in the fridge when we were kiddos. I used to love it slathered with jelly—weird maybe, but I gotta be me.

MAKES 12+

½ cup (55 g) blanched almond flour

¼ cup (40 g) brown rice flour

¼ cup (30 g) sorghum flour

1 tablespoon caraway seeds

¼ teaspoon baking powder

¼ teaspoon sea salt

1 tablespoon chilled unrefined coconut oil

2 tablespoons cold water, plus more if needed

1 teaspoon cocoa/cacao powder

1 teaspoon blackstrap molasses

1. Preheat the oven to 375°F (190°C). Cut two baking-sheet-sized pieces of unbleached parchment paper; set aside.

2. In a bowl using a fork, or in a food processor fitted with the S-blade, mix together the flours, caraway seeds, baking powder, and salt. Cut the oil into the flour mixture until uniformly crumbly, then add 2 tablespoons of the cold water until crumbles start to stick together. Use your hands to form a ball of dough. If it's too dry, add 1 teaspoon water at a time until the dough forms a ball, but note: Less is more; work the dough with your hands first.

3. Cut the dough ball in half and roll one half into a 1- to 2-inch (2.5 to 5 cm) wide snake shape; set aside. Work the cacao powder and molasses into the other dough half with the fork and roll into a "snake" as well. Twist the two together lengthwise and then roll into a ball, maintaining the swirl effect.

4. Place the dough ball on one piece of parchment paper and lay the other sheet on top. Use a rolling pin to flatten to ⅛ inch (3 mm) between the sheets. Peel back the top sheet and use a knife to sculpt the dough into a rectangle, or leave the edges rustic—baker's choice—then score cracker shapes and poke holes in each cracker with the tines of a fork. Slide the dough and parchment onto a baking sheet. Bake for 10 to 15 minutes, until the edges begin to brown. Remove from the oven and cool on the baking sheet.

Seeded Onion Crackers

These crackers add flavorful crunch to salads and are
tasty dipped into Apple & Onion Soup (page 180).
Try them with a spread of Cream Cheese (page 128) and
some chopped dates for a taste of heaven.

MAKES 12+

2 tablespoons sunflower seeds

2 teaspoons raw sesame seeds

1 teaspoon raw poppy seeds

1 tablespoon plus ½ teaspoon
chilled unrefined coconut oil

2 tablespoons minced
yellow onion

1 cup (110 g) almond flour

¼ teaspoon baking powder

¼ teaspoon sea salt

¼ teaspoon fresh-cracked
black pepper

1 tablespoon cold water,
plus more if needed

1   Preheat the oven to 375°F (190°C). Cut two baking-sheet-sized pieces of
    unbleached parchment paper; set one aside and line a baking sheet with
    the other. Scatter the sunflower, sesame, and poppy seeds on the baking
    sheet and toast for 3 to 5 minutes. Remove from the oven and set the lined
    baking sheet aside.

2   In a skillet heated to medium, add ½ teaspoon of the oil and sauté the
    onion for 3 to 5 minutes, until the onion starts to brown; remove from
    the heat and toss into a large mixing bowl. Add the almond flour, toasted
    seeds, baking powder, salt, and pepper to the bowl; stir together. Cut the
    remaining 1 tablespoon oil into the flour mixture until uniformly crumbly.
    Add 1 tablespoon of the cold water until crumbles start to stick together.
    Use your hands to try to form a ball of dough. If it's too dry, add 1 teaspoon
    water at a time until the dough forms a ball, but note: Less is more; work
    the dough well with your hands first.

3   Place the dough ball on one piece of parchment paper and lay the other
    sheet on top. Use a rolling pin to flatten to ⅛ inch (3 mm) between the
    sheets. Peel back the top sheet and use a knife to sculpt the dough into a
    rectangle, or leave the edges rustic—baker's choice—then score cracker
    shapes and poke holes in each cracker with the tines of a fork. Slide the
    dough and parchment onto the baking sheet. Bake for 10 to 12 minutes,
    until the edges begin to brown. Remove from the oven and cool on the
    baking sheet.

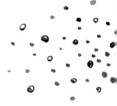

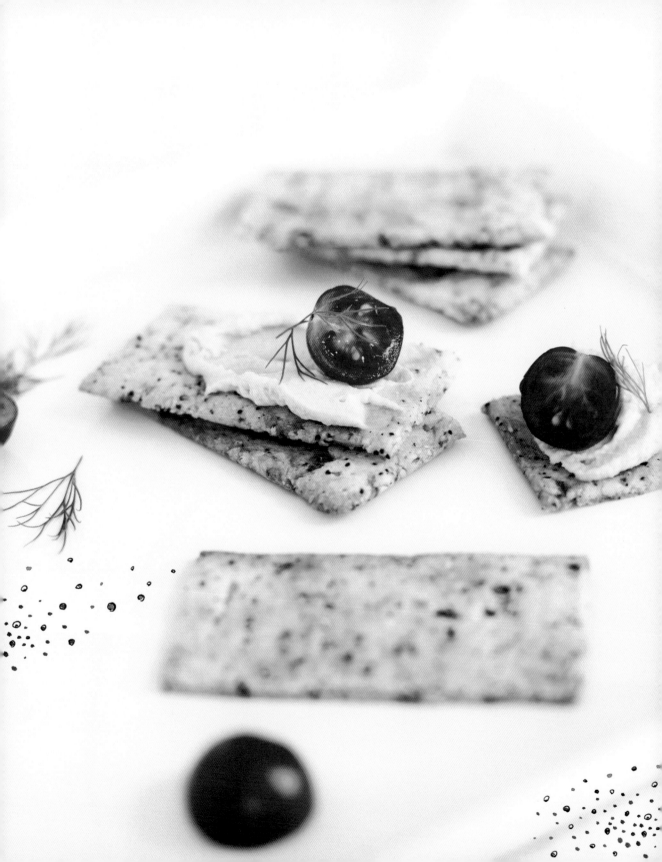

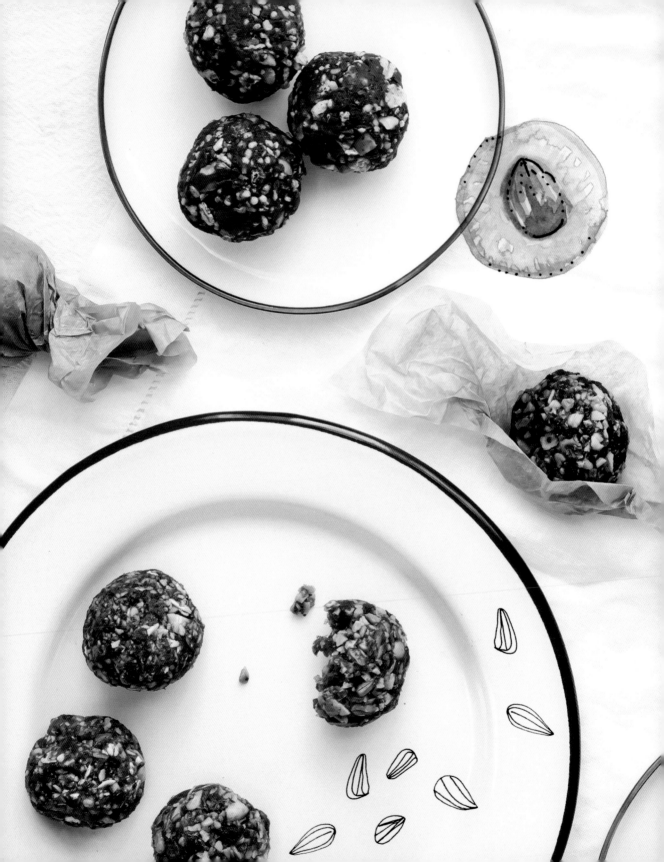

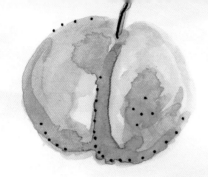

Amazeballs

By simply combining some natural sticky sweetness with a few whole food ingredients, you get a tasty on-the-go protein popper that travels easily and keeps in the fridge for weeks and the freezer for months. Try spicy chipotle and honey, or pumpkin spice and pecan—the possible sweet and savory combinations are infinite.

If you'd like additional texture or flavor on the outside of your Amazeballs, dust them with cacao powder or roll them in toasted and chopped nuts, seeds, and/or shredded coconut. Try a drizzle or dip into melted chocolate and chill. OK, I'll stop now.

Amazeball combos clockwise from top left:
Cacao, cayenne, cinnamon & almond; Honey Mustard (page 127);
cranberry, nutmeg & walnut.

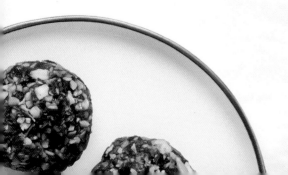

Amazeballs

MAKES 16
PREP TIME: 10 TO 15 MINUTES

This template calls for rolling these snacks into little balls, but feel free to press them into a pan, chill, and then cut into any shape you like for "bars." When storing in the fridge or freezer, layer them with a piece of unbleached parchment paper so they don't stick together. Try to source organic, preservative- and sulfite-free, unsweetened or naturally sweetened dried fruits. If your dried fruit is a bit too dry, soak it in some water until plump again. If your final mixture is too sticky, add some dryness with oats or nuts. If it's not sticky enough, add more dates— you know where I'm going with this—freestyle. Pretoast nuts, seeds, and coconut for extra flavor.

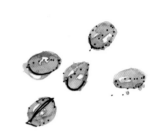

What you need no matter what:

¼ teaspoon sea salt, plus more to taste

2 to 3 teaspoons unrefined coconut oil, gently warmed to liquid (optional)

1 In a food processor, pulse together Big Texture, Tiny Texture (if using), and the **salt** 25 to 30 times, until well mixed but maintaining pea-sized texture.

Big Texture ---- *and/or* ----> Tiny Texture

1 CUP TOTAL
Choose one or combine; all raw, unsalted

Almonds   Pecans

Brazil nuts   Pepitas

Cashews   Pine nuts

Hazelnuts   Sunflower seeds

Macadamia nuts   Walnuts

¼ CUP TOTAL
Choose one or combine, or skip altogether

Poppy seeds

Sesame seeds

Chia seeds

Hemp seeds

2 Add Flavor and Special Additions (if using) and pulse 5 to 10 more times, until the ingredients are evenly distributed, but you still maintain larger pieces for textural variation.

Flavor Optional

Choose any of these in combination for sweet OR - → *Choose any of these in combination for savory*

½ to 1 teaspoon extract (almond, chocolate, mint, hazelnut, vanilla)

¼ to 1 teaspoon ground cinnamon

¼ to ½ teaspoon ground cardamom

1 to 2 teaspoons grated citrus zest

2 to 3 teaspoons ground tea leaves (any)

1 tablespoon ground coffee

1 to 4 teaspoons chopped fresh herbs (thyme, basil, mint)

1 to 6 teaspoons cocoa/cacao powder

1 tablespoon pumpkin pie spice

1 teaspoon ground allspice

Pinch ground cloves

1 teaspoon minced onion

1 small garlic clove, minced

¼ to 1 teaspoon paprika (regular or smoked)

¼ to 1 teaspoon ground coriander

¼ to 1 teaspoon ground cumin

½ to 1 teaspoon grated citrus zest

¼ to ½ teaspoon liquid smoke

1 to 4 teaspoons chopped fresh herbs (rosemary, thyme, sage, chives, oregano, basil)

¼ to 1 teaspoon fresh-cracked black pepper

1 to 3 teaspoons cocoa/cacao powder

1 to 2 teaspoons whole-grain or Dijon mustard

¼ to 1 teaspoon chipotle powder

Special Additions

Choose one or combine, or skip altogether

¼ cup (30 g) shredded carrot

¼ to ½ cup (30 to 60 g) dried fruit

¼ cup (20 g) rolled oats

¼ to ½ cup (20 to 40 g) shredded or flaked coconut

1 to 2 tablespoons Sucanat

1 to 2 tablespoons raw, unpasteurized honey

¼ to ½ cup (45 to 90 g) chocolate chips

1 to 2 tablespoons nut/seed butter (almond, tahini, cashew, pecan)

¼ to ½ cup (8 to 15 g) crispy brown rice cereal

---

3 Add Stickiness and the **oil** (if using; nice for buttery smoothness) and pulse 10 to 15 more times, until everything sticks together. Don't overprocess; you don't want paste! You want texture. Season with more salt if you like. Roll 1 tablespoon of the mixture at a time with your hands into a ball. Repeat until all the mix is used. Chill for at least 1 hour.

Stickiness

1 TO 1¼ CUP TOTAL
Choose one or combine

Dates, pitted (Medjool and Deglet Noor are nice and sticky; my fave binder)

Dried apricots

Raisins (any kind)

Dried figs

Dried prunes

Dried cherries

Caramel-Cocoa Crunch Amazeballs

These are one of my favorite treats when I want something sweet that also has a load of nutrition. They're great for snacking on a long hike or bike ride—energy and protein in each bite. Wanna officially make them dessert? Dip them in a melted 3-ounce (85 g) dairy-free chocolate bar and chill like truffles.

MAKES 16

¼ cup (35 g) raw, unsalted almonds

¼ cup (35 g) raw, unsalted cashews

¼ cup (25 g) raw, unsalted pecans

¼ cup (25 g) raw, unsalted walnuts

Pinch plus ¼ teaspoon sea salt, plus more to taste

2 tablespoons cocoa/cacao powder

1 tablespoon Sucanat

1 teaspoon vanilla extract

1 cup (150 g) packed pitted Medjool dates

2 teaspoons unrefined coconut oil

½ cup (15 g) crispy brown rice cereal

1. Preheat the oven to 350°F (180°C). Line a baking sheet with unbleached parchment paper and spread the almonds, cashews, pecans, and walnuts in one layer on the sheet so they have room to roast mostly untouched on all sides. Sprinkle with the pinch of salt and pop in the oven for 7 minutes. Remove from the baking sheet and toss in the food processor.

2. Add the cocoa powder, Sucanat, vanilla extract, and the ¼ teaspoon salt—pulse 5 to 10 times, until everything starts to break up and mix together.

3. Add the dates and oil and pulse 5 to 7 more times, until everything sticks together. Don't overprocess; you don't want paste! Sprinkle in the brown rice cereal and pulse together 1 to 3 times to simply incorporate. Season with more salt if you like and pulse 3 to 5 more times.

4. Roll 1 tablespoon of the mixture at a time with your hands into a 1½ to 2-inch (4 to 5 cm) ball. Repeat until all the mix is used. Chill for 1 hour.

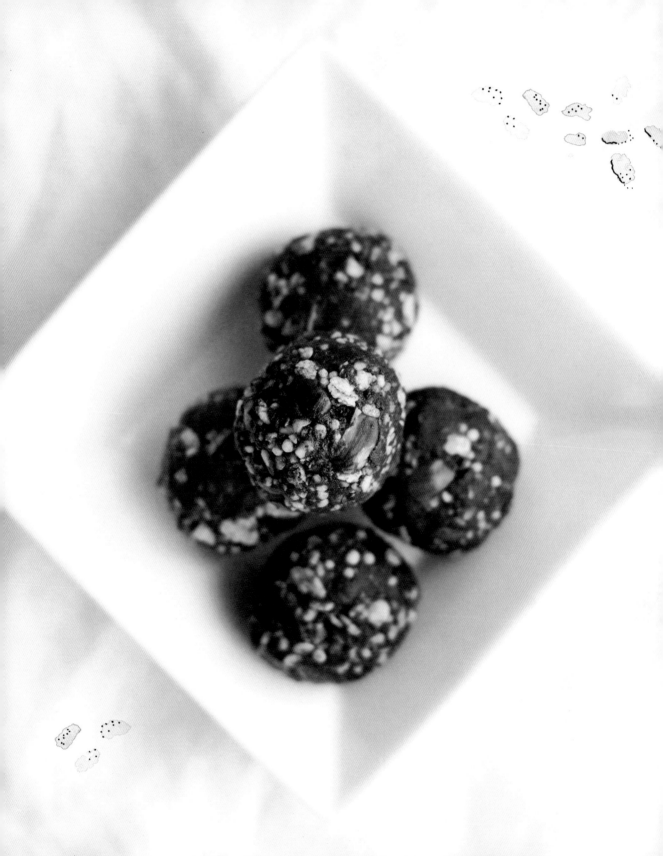

Apricot & Salted Sunflower Seed Amazeballs

A simple, smells-so-good popper—a mix of toasted goodness like nuts, seeds, and coconut with sticky-sweet apricots, raisins, and some orange zest for good measure.

MAKES 16

½ cup (70 g) raw, unsalted sunflower seeds

¼ cup (35 g) raw, unsalted almonds

¼ cup (50 g) raw, unsalted walnuts

Pinch plus ¼ teaspoon sea salt, plus more to taste

½ cup (40 g) flaked coconut

1 teaspoon grated orange zest

½ teaspoon vanilla extract

¼ teaspoon ground cardamom

½ cup (80 g) dried apricots

¼ cup (40 g) dried pineapple

¼ cup (40 g) golden raisins

2 teaspoons unrefined coconut oil

1. Preheat the oven to 350°F (180°C). Line a baking sheet with unbleached parchment paper and spread the sunflower seeds, almonds, and walnuts in one layer on the sheet so they have room to roast mostly untouched on all sides. Sprinkle with the pinch of salt and pop in the oven for 7 minutes. Remove from the baking sheet and toss into the food processor.

2. Spread the coconut flakes on the parchment-lined sheet and toast in the oven for 2 to 3 minutes—keep your eye on it so it doesn't burn—and add to the food processor. Add the ¼ teaspoon salt, orange zest, vanilla extract, and cardamom to the processor; pulse 5 to 10 times, until the ingredients are evenly distributed, but maintain larger pieces for textural variation.

3. Add the apricots, pineapple, raisins, and oil and pulse 5 to 10 more times, until everything sticks together. Don't overprocess; you don't want paste! You want texture. Season with more salt if you like and pulse 3 to 5 more times to incorporate.

4. Roll 1 tablespoon of the mixture at a time with your hands into a 1½ to 2-inch (4 to 5 cm) ball. Repeat until all the mix is used. Chill for 1 hour.

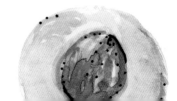

Honey Mustard Amazeballs

These snacks can also have a savory twist—a combo of smoke, sweet, and salt make this honey mustard variation a great example. It just may become your new fave. Be sure to skip pretoasting the hemp seeds—those tasty little babies are sensitive to heat.

MAKES 16

½ cup (70 g) raw, unsalted almonds

¼ cup (30 g) raw, unsalted pepitas

¼ cup (20 g) rolled oats

Pinch plus ¼ teaspoon sea salt, plus more to taste

2¼ teaspoons unrefined coconut oil

1 teaspoon minced onion

1 small garlic clove, minced

1 cup (150 g) pitted Medjool dates

¼ cup (40 g) hemp seeds

1 tablespoon raw honey

2 teaspoons whole-grain mustard

½ teaspoon fresh-cracked black pepper

½ teaspoon grated lemon zest

¼ teaspoon liquid smoke or ¼ teaspoon smoked paprika

1. Preheat the oven to 350°F (180°C). Line a baking sheet with unbleached parchment paper and spread the almonds, pepitas, and oats in one layer on the sheet so they have room to roast. Sprinkle with the pinch of salt and pop in the oven for 7 minutes. Remove from the baking sheet and toss in the food processor.

2. In a small sauté pan heated to medium, add ¼ teaspoon of the oil and sauté the onion and garlic for 5 minutes, then add to the food processor. Add the dates, hemp seeds, honey, mustard, pepper, zest, the ¼ teaspoon salt, the remaining 2 teaspoons oil, and liquid smoke; pulse 5 to 10 times, until everything starts to stick together. Don't overprocess; you don't want paste—you want texture. Season with more salt if you like and pulse 3 to 5 more times to incorporate.

3. Roll 1 tablespoon of the mixture at a time with your hands into a 1½ to 2-inch (4 to 5 cm) ball. Repeat until all the mix is used. Chill for 1 hour.

Learn more about the benefits,
safety, and possibilities of fermented foods:
yumuniverse.com/?s=fermented

Probiotic
Cream
Cheese

Making dairy-free, probiotic-rich cream cheese
at home is easy—you just need 1 to 3 days of fermentation
time, so plan ahead. Cashews make the creamiest
base, so I call for using them 100 percent or mixed with
other nuts or seeds for velvety texture and most
"cream cheese" flavor.

Don't freak if walnuts or pecans turn purple,
or sunflower seeds darken—pigments in them
are simply reacting to the pH of the cheese—
they're safe to eat!

For best results, use raw, organic ingredients
and a refrigerated probiotic capsule.
A 1- to 2-day ferment is plenty of time to get
some zing. The longer you ferment, the
more sour and "funky" or "fragrant"—
like a fine cheese! Let your nose and taste buds
decide what's the best flavor for you.

Cream Cheese combos on this page (clockwise from left): Cashew-honey cream cheese,
smoked paprika & toasted mixed nuts; spicy cashew-almond cream cheese
with roasted jalapeño & poblano peppers; walnut & cashew "blue cheese" swirl.

10 TO 20 SERVINGS
PREP TIME: 5 TO 15 MINUTES
FERMENTATION TIME 1 TO 3 DAYS

What you need no matter what:

1½ cups (210 g) raw, unsalted cashews, soaked for 4 to 6 hours

1 cup (240 ml) water, plus more for soaking

1 probiotic capsule (the clear kind with two see-through halves you can open)

½ teaspoon sea salt

1 Place the soaked **cashews,** Base, and **water** into the blender and mix until ultra-smooth, adding 1 tablespoon water at a time if needed to reach a creamy, melted-ice-cream consistency. Cream cheese will lose 10 to 15 percent water volume as it ferments the next few days—it will firm up.

Base

½ CUP TOTAL
Choose one (page 10 for soaking tips); all raw, unsalted

Cashews, soaked for 4 to 6 hours

Almonds, soaked for 8 to 12 hours

Sunflower seeds, soaked for 8 to 12 hours

Walnuts, soaked for 8 to 12 hours

Macadamia nuts, not soaked

Pecans, soaked for 8 to 12 hours

2 Transfer the mixture to a clean glass bowl using a nonmetal spoon. Stir the contents of the **probiotic capsule** and the **salt** into the mixture. Cover with a cheesecloth and secure with a rubber band. Place in a warm spot in the kitchen out of sunlight for 1 to 3 days. Use a clean utensil to sample after day 1—let it ferment a few more days until the desired sourness is achieved (taste daily).

3 Once sour enough, stir in Sweet and Fold-Ins (if using). Store in an airtight glass container in the fridge for 2 to 4 weeks—it will continue to ferment/sour at a slower pace.

Sweet --> Fold-Ins

1 TO 3
TABLESPOONS
TOTAL
Choose one or skip

Raw, unpasteurized honey

Maple syrup

Sucanat

Coconut sugar

Choose as many as you like, or skip altogether

1 teaspoon extract (for sweet cheese: almond, vanilla)

1 tablespoon seeds (caraway, fennel, poppy, sesame)

¼ to 1 teaspoon ground cinnamon

½ to 1 teaspoon grated citrus zest or juice

¼ cup (25 g) chopped sun-dried tomatoes

1 to 4 teaspoons chopped fresh herbs

1 tablespoon dulse flakes

¼ to 1 teaspoon fresh-cracked black pepper

1 to 2 teaspoons nutritional yeast

1 to 3 teaspoons seasoning mix (ranch, taco, herbes de Provence)

1 to 3 garlic cloves, minced

¼ cup (35 g) nuts & seeds, toasted, chopped

¼ cup (40 g) chopped onion or shallot, raw or sautéed

Dried fruit (raisins, dates, cherries)

½ to 1 cup (55 to 110 g) minced veggies

1 to 2 teaspoons miso

Garden Veggie Cream Cheese

Infuse some serious color and flavor into homemade cream cheese with vibrant veggies like red pepper, carrot, and scallions. Spread some on homemade Crackers (page 112) or whisk some together with some water, a squeeze of lemon juice, and olive oil for a creamy salad dressing. Remember, this recipe requires 1 to 3 days of fermentation time, so plan ahead!

10 TO 20 SERVINGS

2 cups (280 g) raw, unsalted cashews, soaked for 4 to 6 hours

1 cup (240 ml) water

1 probiotic capsule

½ teaspoon sea salt, plus more to taste

½ teaspoon coconut oil

¼ cup (40 g) diced shallot

1 garlic clove, minced

¼ cup (25 g) diced celery

¼ cup (40 g) diced red bell pepper

¼ cup (25 g) diced scallions

¼ cup (30 g) diced, shredded, or chopped carrots

1 tablespoon chopped fresh chives

½ teaspoon grated lemon zest

¼ teaspoon fresh-cracked black pepper

1. Drain the cashews and rinse well, then mix with the water in a blender until ultra-smooth. Cream cheese will lose 10 to 15 percent water volume as it ferments the next few days. It will firm up.

2. Transfer the mixture to a clean glass bowl using a nonmetal spoon. Open up the probiotic capsule, sprinkle the contents into the cheese, add the salt, and stir. Cover with a cheesecloth and secure with a rubber band. Place in a warm spot in the kitchen out of sunlight for 1 to 3 days. Use a clean utensil to sample after day 1; if it tastes good to you, it's done. If you want more sourness, let it ferment another 1 to 2 days, until the desired flavor is achieved.

3. In a pan heated to medium, add the oil and sauté the shallot for 5 minutes, then add the garlic and stir together for 3 minutes. When it starts to brown, remove from the heat and fold into your cream cheese with the celery, red pepper, scallions, carrots, chives, zest, black pepper, and more salt if needed. Chill and serve.

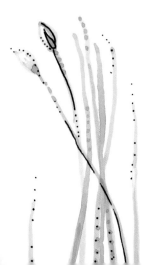

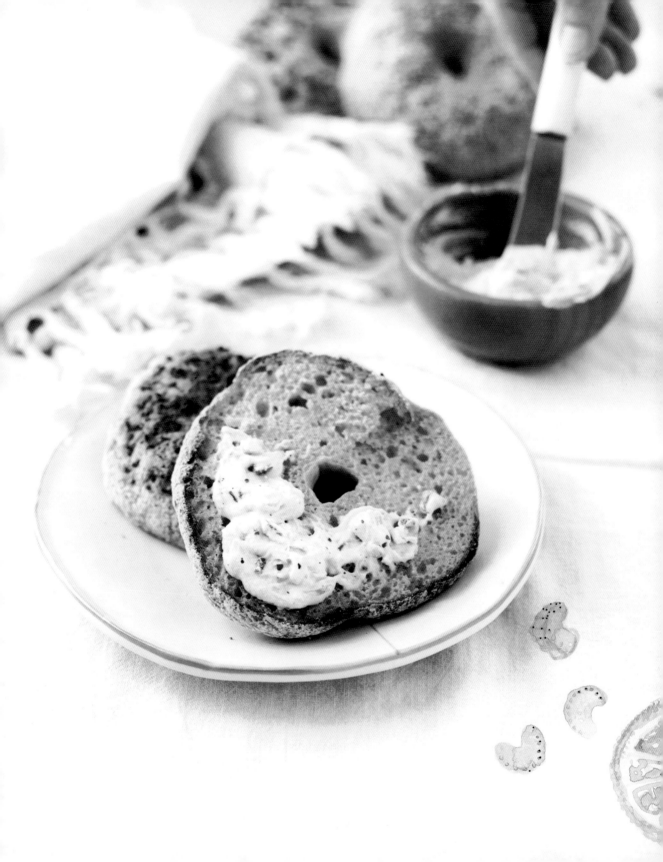

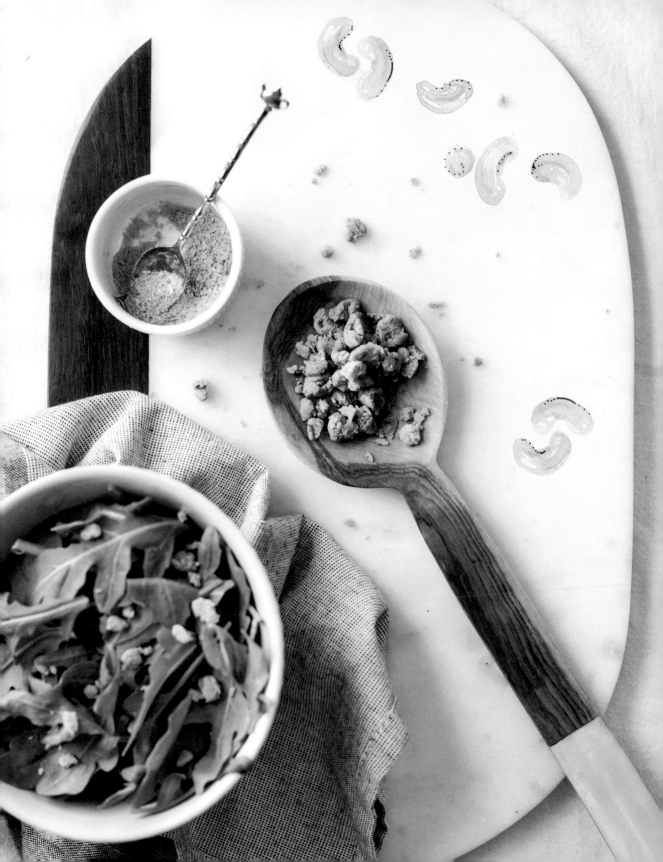

Cashew-Almond Cheese Crumbles

A staple for topping salads and tacos—delicious in a savory Muffin (page 63). Use a low-temp oven setting or a dehydrator to dry the crumbles.

While not called for in this recipe, if you want more "funk" to resemble feta or blue cheese, add ½ to 1 teaspoon apple cider vinegar and/or lemon juice to taste. If you use pecans or walnuts instead of almonds, you'll get some purple hues, à la blue cheese.

10 TO 20 SERVINGS

1½ cups (210 g) raw, unsalted cashews, soaked for 4 to 6 hours

½ cup (70 g) raw, unsalted almonds, soaked for 8 to 12 hours

1 cup (240 ml) water

1 probiotic capsule

½ teaspoon sea salt, plus more to taste

2 teaspoons chickpea miso (or any miso you like)

2 teaspoons nutritional yeast

Two pinches Sucanat or coconut sugar (optional)

1. Drain the cashews and almonds and rinse. Place the nuts and water in a blender and mix until ultra-smooth. Cream cheese will lose 10 to 15 percent water volume as it ferments. It will firm up.

2. Transfer the mixture to a glass bowl using a nonmetal spoon. Open the probiotic capsule, sprinkle the contents into the cheese, add the salt, and stir. Cover with a dish towel and secure with a rubber band. Place in a warm spot in the kitchen out of sunlight for 1 to 3 days. Use a clean utensil to sample after day 1; if it tastes good to you, it's done. Want more sourness? Let it ferment another 1 to 2 days to taste.

3. Preheat the oven to 225°F (105°C). Fold together the cheese, miso, nutritional yeast, more sea salt a pinch at a time if needed, and Sucanat (if using; it helps round out flavors). Spread the cheese ¼ inch (6 mm) thick on a piece of unbleached parchment paper or a silicone baking mat and dry in the oven for 30 to 40 minutes, until the top and edges are dry to the touch, but still soft like goat cheese crumbles. Remove from the oven and cool on the baking sheet. Chill, crumble, and serve.

Honey & Toasted Almond Cream Cheese

At my very first design job in Chicago, I was introduced
to the Monday morning meeting with bagels and cream cheese.
But not the kind of silver-plastic-tub cream cheese
I grew up with; this stuff was downright artisanal, sweetened
with honey and loaded with crunchy toasted almonds.
After the first bite, it was committed to memory forever, and
now I'm sharing my simple, dairy-free riff with you.

10 TO 20 SERVINGS

1½ cups (210 g) raw, unsalted cashews, soaked for 4 to 6 hours

¾ cup (105 g) raw, unsalted almonds, ½ cup (70 g) soaked for 8 to 12 hours

1 cup (240 ml) water

1 probiotic capsule

½ teaspoon plus pinch sea salt, plus more to taste

3 tablespoons raw, unpasteurized honey

1. Drain the soaked cashews and almonds and rinse well. Place the soaked nuts and water in a blender and mix until ultra-smooth. Cream cheese will lose 10 to 15 percent water volume as it ferments the next few days. It will firm up.

2. Transfer the mixture to a clean glass bowl using a nonmetal spoon. Open up the probiotic capsule, sprinkle the contents into the cheese, add the salt, and stir. Cover with a cheesecloth and secure with a rubber band. Place in a warm spot in the kitchen out of sunlight for 1 to 3 days. Use a clean utensil to sample after day 1; if it tastes good to you, it's done. If you want more sourness, let it ferment another 1 to 2 days, until desired flavor is achieved.

3. Preheat the oven to 350°F (180°C). Chop the remaining ¼ cup unsoaked almonds. Line a baking sheet with unbleached parchment paper and spread the chopped almonds in one layer on the sheet so they have room to roast mostly untouched on all sides. Sprinkle with the pinch of salt and pop in the oven for 7 minutes. Fold the chopped almonds into the cream cheese with the honey and more sea salt if you like. Chill and serve.

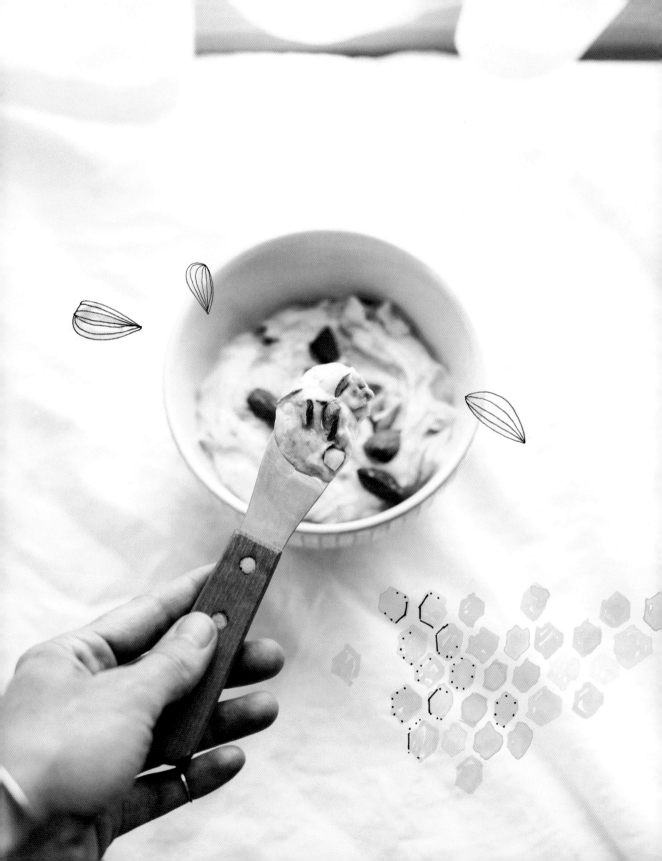

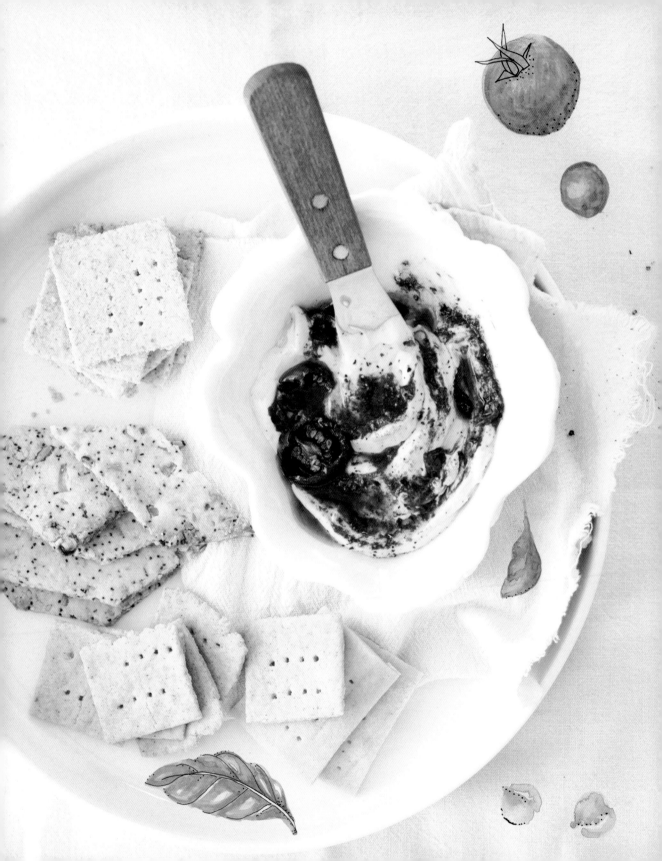

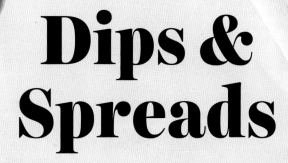

Dips & Spreads

Dips and spreads are very similar—the biggest difference is the thickness. If it takes a knife to slather it on a cracker, it's a spread. If you can plunge a stalk of celery in it, it's a dip. Both are ridiculously easy to make, and the variations are plantiful. Serve them chilled, or quick-broil them for a warm, comforting snack.

When serving, swirl in extras like Supergreen Pesto (page 33), harissa, honey, Chimichurri (page 30), or olive oil—top with toasted nuts, seeds, herbs, and fresh-cracked black pepper. Keep at least one dip or spread in the fridge each week, and you'll be more inclined to snack on healthy goodies. They also add great flavor to a Wrap (page 217).

Spread combo shown here:
Yogurt-chickpea dip with Supergreen Pesto (page 33),
roasted cherry tomatoes & extra virgin olive oil.

Dips & Spreads

When using veggies in your dip, try them raw or roast, caramelize, or char them on the grill for extra flavor. Also, season to taste!

12+ SERVINGS
PREP TIME: 15 TO 35 MINUTES

What you need no matter what:

1 tablespoon water, plus more as needed

½ to 1 teaspoon sea salt

1 Place Base 1 and Base 2 into the blender or food processor and purée. Add the **water** 1 tablespoon at a time to the blender if needed to reach the smooth consistency you want for a dip or spread—note before you do, you may be adding Oil (a.k.a. liquid) in Step 2.

Base 1 ----- *and* ---→ Base 2

1 CUP TOTAL
Choose one

Coconut Yogurt
(page 94)

Raw, unsalted
sunflower seeds,
soaked

Raw, unsalted
cashews, soaked

Probiotic Cream
Cheese (page 128)

Coconut cream
(skimmed from the
top of a chilled can
of coconut milk)

2 CUPS TOTAL
Choose one
or combine

Coconut Yogurt
(page 94)

Raw, unsalted
cashews, soaked
for 4 to 6 hours

Probiotic Cream
Cheese (page 128)

Beans or legumes,
cooked (any kind)

Winter squash,
roasted or steamed
(any kind)

Roots, roasted or
steamed (any kind)

Chopped avocado

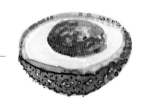

2 Add Flavor (if using), Oil (if using), and Acid and blend long enough to incorporate, but quick enough that you maintain colorful specks from herbs and spices.

Flavor

Choose one or combine or skip altogether

¼ to ½ teaspoon
chipotle powder

½ to 1 teaspoon
garam masala

1 to 3 teaspoons
nutritional yeast

1 to 3 teaspoons
tahini

¼ to 1 teaspoon
ground cinnamon

½ to 1 teaspoon
ground cumin

½ to 1 teaspoon
ground coriander

1 to 4 teaspoons
chopped fresh herbs
(rosemary, thyme,
sage, dill, chives,
oregano, basil,
parsley, cilantro)

¼ to ½ teaspoon
cayenne pepper

½ to 2 teaspoons
paprika (smoked
or plain)

¼ to 1 teaspoon
liquid smoke

Pinch to ¼ teaspoon
ground cardamom

Oil ------------ *and/or* ----------→ Acid

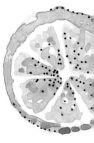

¼ CUP (60 ML) TOTAL
Choose one or skip altogether

Extra virgin olive oil   Sunflower seed oil

Grapeseed oil   Pumpkin seed oil

Avocado oil   Roasted/toasted oils
(hazelnut, walnut,
pecan, sesame)

1 TO 3 TEASPOONS
Choose one

Citrus juice
(lemon, lime)

Vinegar (apple
cider, red wine,
balsamic)

---

3 Transfer the mixture to a large bowl and stir together with Fold-Ins (if using)
and the **salt** to taste.

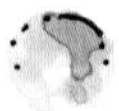

Fold-Ins

Choose one or combine, or skip altogether; chop, slice, or dice

¼ to ½ cup (30 to
60 g) dried fruit

½ to 1 cup packed
dark greens

¼ cup (25 g)
sun-dried tomatoes

¼ to ½ cup (60 to
120 ml) salsa

½ to 1 teaspoon
grated citrus zest

¼ cup (35 g)
capers/olives

¼ cup (20 g)
jalapeños

1 cup (260 g)
marinated
artichoke hearts

¼ to 1 cup (25 to
100 g) scallions

¼ to ½ cup
(25 to 100 g) celery

¼ to 1 cup (35 to
145 g) fresh corn
kernels (non-GMO)

¼ to ½ cup
(35 to 150 g) bell
pepper (any)

¼ to ½ cup
(45 to 90 g)
Cashew-Almond
Cheese Crumbles
(page 133)

¼ to ½ cup (40 to
160 g) onions or
shallots, caramelized

¼ to ½ cup
(35 to 150 g)
cherry tomatoes

¼ to ½ cup (35 to
145 g) fresh peas

¼ to ½ cup roots,
diced and roasted
or shredded raw
(beet, carrot)

¼ to ½ cup (25 to
45 g) fennel bulb

1 to 3 garlic
cloves, minced

---

4 When serving, drizzle or sprinkle Toppings (if using) onto the dip.
Store in the fridge for 1 to 2 weeks.

Toppings: Sprinkle/Swirl

Choose one or combine, or skip altogether

Fresh-cracked
black pepper

Scallions, sliced

Fresh herbs, chopped

Fresh lemon juice

Toasted nuts or seeds
(any kind), chopped

Extra oil from step 2

Raw, unpasteurized
honey

Nuts & seeds,
toasted, chopped
(any)

Supergreen
Pesto (page 33)

Chimichurri
(page 30)

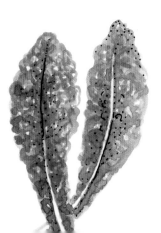

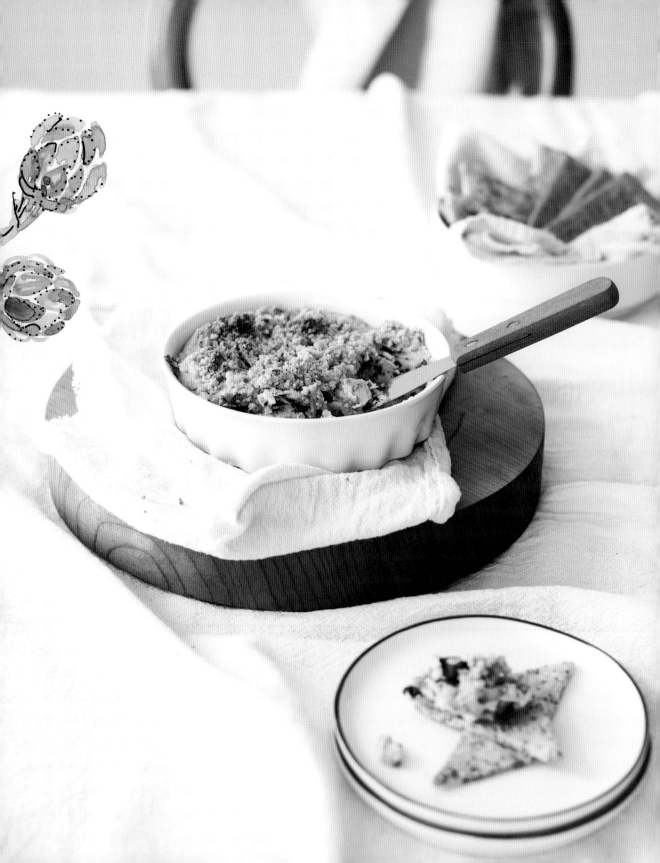

Warm Tuscan Kale & Artichoke Dip

A simple freestyle from a classic recipe—reenvisioned sans dairy. I bet no one you serve it to will notice. They'll be too busy raving about how tasty it is. If you can't find Tuscan (lacinato) kale, don't let that stop you—use whatever kind you can find.

12+ SERVINGS

¼ cup (30 g) blanched almond flour

1 tablespoon unrefined coconut oil

¾ teaspoon sea salt, plus more to taste

3 cups (420 g) raw, unsalted cashews, soaked for 4 to 6 hours

2 cups (480 ml) water

1 tablespoon fresh lemon juice

1 teaspoon grated lemon zest

¼ to ½ teaspoon cayenne pepper

1 cup (260 g) marinated artichoke hearts, drained and chopped

1 cup (15 g) packed lacinato kale, chopped into tiny pieces

¼ cup (25 g) sliced scallions (2 to 3 stalks)

Fresh-cracked black pepper

1. In a small bowl, use a fork to cut together the flour, oil, and a few pinches of salt until crumbly; set aside.

2. Combine the soaked cashews, water, lemon juice, lemon zest, ¾ teaspoon of the salt, and the cayenne to taste in a blender and purée until silky smooth. Transfer to a mixing bowl and fold together with the artichoke hearts, kale, scallions, and black pepper to taste. Season with more salt if you like.

3. Transfer to a 6- to 8-inch (15 to 20 cm) ceramic or glass baking dish, evenly distribute the flour mixture so it covers the entire top of the dip, and sprinkle with a few grinds of black pepper. Turn the broiler to high and broil the top of the dip for 2 to 3 minutes, until browned. Allow to cool for 5 to 10 minutes and serve warm.

4. Store in an airtight glass container in the fridge for 1 to 2 weeks and enjoy chilled or rewarmed from the oven.

Cinnamon-Spiced Red Lentil Dip

This is a flavor-packed, protein-powered dip that's great with raw veggies, and extra special with roasted almonds and a drizzle of honey.

12+ SERVINGS

Handful almonds (optional)

¼ cup (60 ml) extra virgin olive oil, plus more for a light sauté and serving

1 cup (160 g) chopped yellow onion

2 cups (400 g) cooked red lentils (roughly ¾ cup/145 g dry; see page 11)

1 cup (220 g) coconut cream (skimmed from the top of a chilled can of coconut milk)

½ cup (75 g) golden raisins, plus more for garnish

1 teaspoon apple cider vinegar

½ teaspoon garam masala

½ teaspoon ground cinnamon, plus more to taste

½ teaspoon ground cumin

½ teaspoon sea salt, plus more to taste

Pinch ground cardamom

1 tablespoon water, or more if needed

Raw, unpasteurized honey (optional)

1. If you'd like to top your dip with roasted almonds, preheat the oven to 350°F (180°C) and line a baking sheet with unbleached parchment paper. Roast the almonds for 7 to 10 minutes, until brown and smelling incredible—chop and set aside.

2. In a skillet heated to medium-low, add a drizzle of olive oil and sauté the onion for 7 to 10 minutes, until the onion starts to brown. Remove from the heat and transfer to a blender or food processor.

3. Add the lentils, coconut cream, raisins, ¼ cup (60 ml) oil, vinegar, garam masala, cinnamon, cumin, salt, and cardamom to the blender—purée until silky smooth. Add the water and more salt if needed. Transfer to a serving bowl, drizzle with oil and honey (if using), sprinkle with a pinch of salt, cinnamon, some whole raisins, and the roasted almonds (if using), and serve. Store in an airtight glass container in the fridge for 1 to 2 weeks.

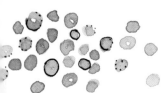

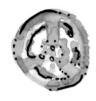

The Best Black Bean Dip

This is a staple recipe that is insanely good with blue corn tortilla chips and dippable veggies like celery, peppers, carrots, and radish. Before blending, char the peppers on the grill for incredible depth of flavor, or simply use them raw. Try this dip as a creamy, flavorful spread for Tacos & Wraps (page 217), too—if you eat it by the spoonful, I won't judge.

12+ SERVINGS

2 cups (340 g) cooked black beans (roughly ¾ cup/145 g dry; see page 11)

½ cup (75 g) diced avocado

½ cup (75 g) chopped red bell pepper

½ cup (110 g) unsweetened Coconut Yogurt (page 94 or store-bought), plus more for garnish

¼ cup (40 g) diced red onion

3 garlic cloves, minced

Handful fresh cilantro, chopped, plus more for garnish

2 tablespoons fresh lime juice

1 tablespoon seeded, chopped jalapeño

1 tablespoon water, or more if needed

1 teaspoon ground coriander

1 teaspoon ground cumin

½ teaspoon sea salt, plus more to taste

¼ teaspoon chipotle powder

Pinch cayenne pepper

Fresh-cracked black pepper to taste

½ cup (75 g) cherry tomatoes, quartered, plus a few more for garnish

1. Combine the beans, avocado, bell pepper, yogurt, onion, garlic, cilantro, lime juice, jalapeño, water, coriander, cumin, salt, chipotle powder, cayenne, and a few grinds of black pepper in a food processor and purée until smooth. Add more salt and black pepper if needed, then fold in the tomatoes.

2. Transfer to a serving bowl and top with a few more tomatoes and cilantro and a drizzle of yogurt. Grab some chips, Crackers (page 112), or veggies to dip and go to town! Store in an airtight glass container in the fridge for 1 to 2 weeks.

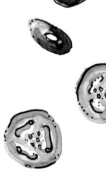

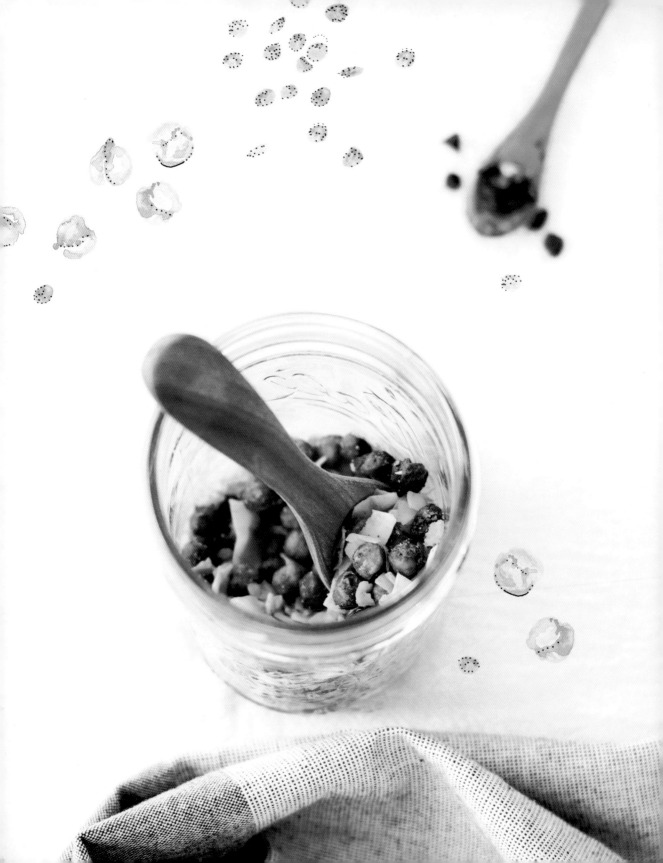

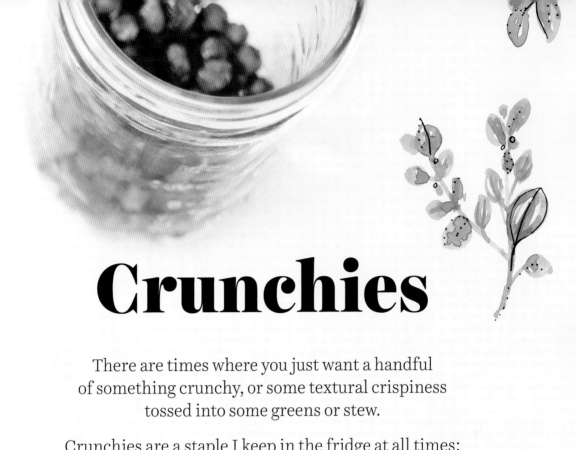

Crunchies

There are times where you just want a handful
of something crunchy, or some textural crispiness
tossed into some greens or stew.

Crunchies are a staple I keep in the fridge at all times;
not only do they add a tasty nutrition, protein, and
crunch boost to salads, soups, and scrambles, they also last
for weeks. Make them sweet or savory—swirl them into
yogurt or eat them as a snack.

Cunchies combos on this spread clockwise from left:
Smoky Coconut Crunch (page 149); harissa & honey chickpeas;
wasabi-lentils & pecans.

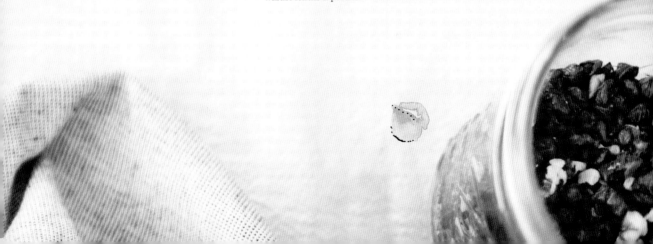

Crunchies

2+ SERVINGS
COOK TIME: 45 TO 55 MINUTES

These can be made simply with Crunch, salt, and pepper, or you can amp them up with exotic spices and herbs. Keep in mind, if you sweeten with a hygroscopic (water-lovin') liquid sweetener like honey, your Crunchies may be softer and stickier once baked.

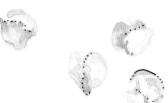

What you need no matter what:

½ **teaspoon sea salt, plus more to taste**

1 Preheat the oven to 350°F (180°C) and line a baking sheet with unbleached parchment paper. Toss together Crunch, Oil, Sweet (if using), and the **salt** until the ingredients are well distributed.

Crunch ----------- *and* -----------→ Oil

2 CUPS TOTAL
Choose one or combine;
see page 11 for cooking tips

Chickpeas, cooked

Lentils (not red—use French, green, brown, or beluga), cooked

2 TO 3 TABLESPOONS TOTAL
Choose one

Avocado oil

Grapeseed oil

Coconut oil, gently warmed to liquid

Sweet

1 TO 6 TEASPOONS TOTAL
Choose one or skip altogether

Raw, unpasteurized honey

Maple syrup

Sucanat

Coconut sugar

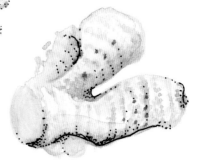

2   Fold in Flavor (if using) until thoroughly coated and spread the mixture in one layer on the baking sheet. Bake for 35 to 40 minutes giving the sheet a shake once during baking time.

Flavor

Choose any of these in combination or skip altogether **AND/OR** --> *Choose one*

½ to 1 teaspoon extract (almond, chocolate, mint hazelnut, vanilla)

¼ to 1 teaspoon ground cinnamon

¼ to ½ teaspoon ground cardamom

1 to 2 teaspoons grated citrus zest

2 to 3 teaspoons ground tea leaves (any)

1 tablespoon ground coffee

1 to 4 teaspoons chopped fresh herbs (thyme, basil, mint)

1 to 6 teaspoons cocoa/cacao powder

1 tablespoon pumpkin pie spice

1 teaspoon ground allspice

Pinch ground cloves

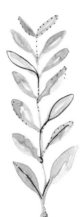

1 to 3 teaspoons za'atar spice blend

1 to 3 teaspoons miso (any)

1 to 3 teaspoons Chinese five-spice

1 to 3 teaspoons BBQ dry rub

1 to 3 teaspoons berbere spice

1 to 3 teaspoons Cajun mix

1 to 3 teaspoons curry powder

1 to 3 teaspoons garam masala

1 to 3 teaspoons Jamaican jerk seasoning

1 to 3 teaspoons Montreal steak seasoning

1 to 3 teaspoons Old Bay Seasoning

1 to 3 teaspoons taco/fajita seasoning mix

3   Remove Crunchies from the oven to fold in any Special Additions (if using). Continue to roast for an additional 10 to 15 minutes until Crunch is crispy and brown.

Special Additions

Choose one or combine, or skip altogether

1 to 2 teaspoons peeled, minced fresh ginger

1 to 2 teaspoons grated citrus zest

¼ to ½ cup (35 to 70 g) raw, unsalted nuts and/or seeds, chopped

1 to 6 garlic cloves, minced

¼ cup (20 g) rolled oats

¼ cup (40 g) hulled buckwheat groats

1 to 4 teaspoons chopped fresh herbs

4   Remove Crunchies from the oven and fold in Finishing Touch (if using). Cool on the baking sheet and season with more salt if needed—Crunchies harden as they cool. Store in the fridge for 2 to 3 weeks.

Finishing Touch

¼ to 1 cup (20 to 85 g) shredded or flaked dried coconut, toasted

1 to 3 teaspoons wasabi powder (choose Flavor wisely if using)

¼ teaspoon liquid smoke

¼ to 1 teaspoon smoked paprika

Choose one or skip altogether

Chinese Five-Spice Lentil & Pecan Crunch

A great snack that also takes an Epic Salad (page 195) with Orange-Sesame Sauce (page 30) to the next level of tasty.

SERVES 8+

2 cups (400 g) cooked lentils (French, green, brown, or beluga; roughly ¾ cup/140 g dry; see page 11)

3 tablespoons grapeseed oil

1 tablespoon Chinese five-spice, to taste

1 tablespoon Sucanat

2 teaspoons coconut aminos (soy sauce or tamari)

2 teaspoons peeled, grated fresh ginger—almost a pulp

½ teaspoon sea salt

Fresh-cracked black pepper

½ cup (50 g) raw, unsalted pecans, chopped very fine

2 garlic cloves, minced

1. Preheat the oven to 350°F (180°C) and line a baking sheet with unbleached parchment paper.

2. In a large bowl, toss together the lentils, oil, five-spice, Sucanat, coconut aminos, ginger, salt, and a few grinds of pepper. Fold together until the lentils are evenly coated. Spread the mixture onto the baking sheet in one layer so everything has room to brown. Bake for 30 minutes, giving the baking sheet a shake every 10 minutes.

3. Remove from the oven and fold in the pecans and garlic. Roast for another 10 minutes until crispy. Allow to cool on the baking sheet—they will harden as they cool. Store in an airtight glass container in the fridge for 2 to 3 weeks.

Smoky Coconut Crunch

If you love a combo of salty, sweet, and smoky, these are your Crunchies (essence of bacon, but not bacon). Make them for the meat eaters in your life to add texture and crunch to salads and snacks. This is a fun one to try on the "coconut haters" out there—it always converts.

SERVES 8+

1 cup (85 g) dry flaked coconut

2 cups (330 g) cooked chickpeas (roughly ¾ cup dry; page 11 for tips)

3 tablespoons unrefined coconut oil

1 teaspoon maple syrup

1 teaspoon grated lemon zest

1 teaspoon smoked paprika

¾ teaspoon sea salt

¼ teaspoon liquid smoke (optional)

1   Preheat the oven to 350°F (180°C) and line a baking sheet with unbleached parchment paper. Sprinkle the coconut evenly on the sheet and toast for 3 minutes. Set aside.

2   In a large bowl, toss together the chickpeas, oil, maple syrup, zest, paprika, and salt. Fold together until the chickpeas are evenly coated. Spread the mixture onto the baking sheet in one layer so they have room to brown. Bake for 40 to 50 minutes, until crispy and brown, giving the baking sheet a shake every 10 minutes.

3   Remove from the oven and allow to cool on the baking sheet—they will harden as they cool. Toss with the toasted coconut and, if you want more smokiness, the liquid smoke. Store in an airtight glass container in the fridge for 2 to 3 weeks.

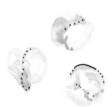
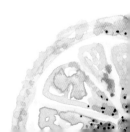

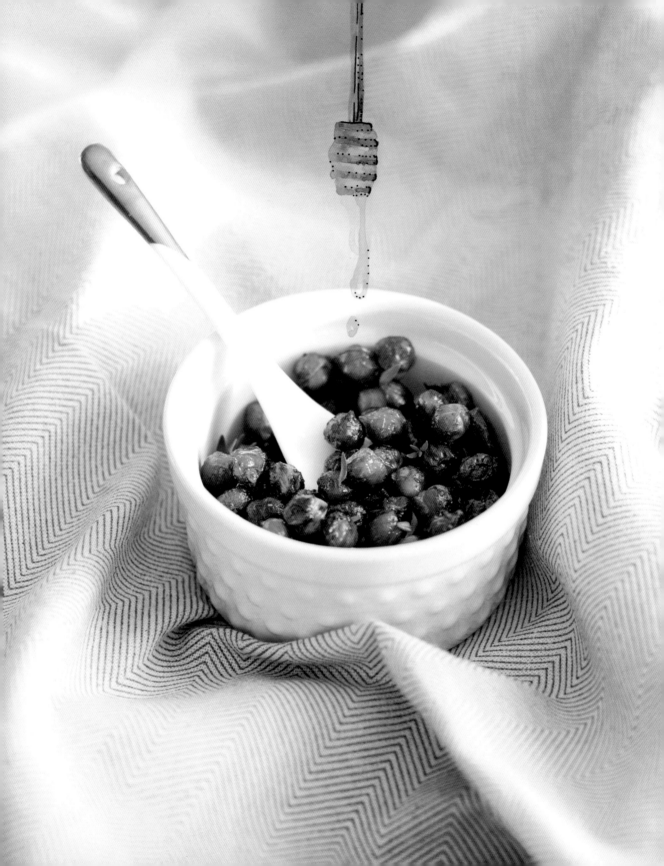

Honey-Roasted Cinnamon & Coriander Chickpeas

I love these little babies swirled into yogurt,
by the handful, and with spring mix or arugula, avocado,
fresh-cracked black pepper, and a simple squeeze
of fresh lemon juice.

SERVES 8+

2 cups (330 g) cooked chickpeas
(roughly ¾ cup/150 g dry;
see page 11)

3 tablespoons unrefined
coconut oil

2 tablespoons raw,
unpasteurized honey

½ teaspoon ground cinnamon

½ teaspoon ground coriander

½ teaspoon sea salt

¼ teaspoon ground cardamom
(optional)

Pinch cayenne pepper
(optional)

1 teaspoon fresh thyme leaves

1   Preheat the oven to 350°F (180°C) and line a baking sheet with unbleached
    parchment paper.

2   In a large bowl, toss together the chickpeas, oil, honey, cinnamon, coriander,
    salt, cardamom, and cayenne. Fold together until the chickpeas are evenly
    coated. Spread the mixture onto the baking sheet in one layer so they have
    room to brown. Bake for 40 minutes, giving the baking sheet a shake every
    10 minutes.

3   Remove from the oven and sprinkle with the thyme; stir to incorporate.
    Roast for another 10 to 15 minutes, until brown. Remove from the oven and
    allow to cool on the baking sheet—they will harden as they cool, but due to
    the moisture in the honey, they may be a bit sticky. Store in an airtight glass
    container in the fridge for 2 to 3 weeks.

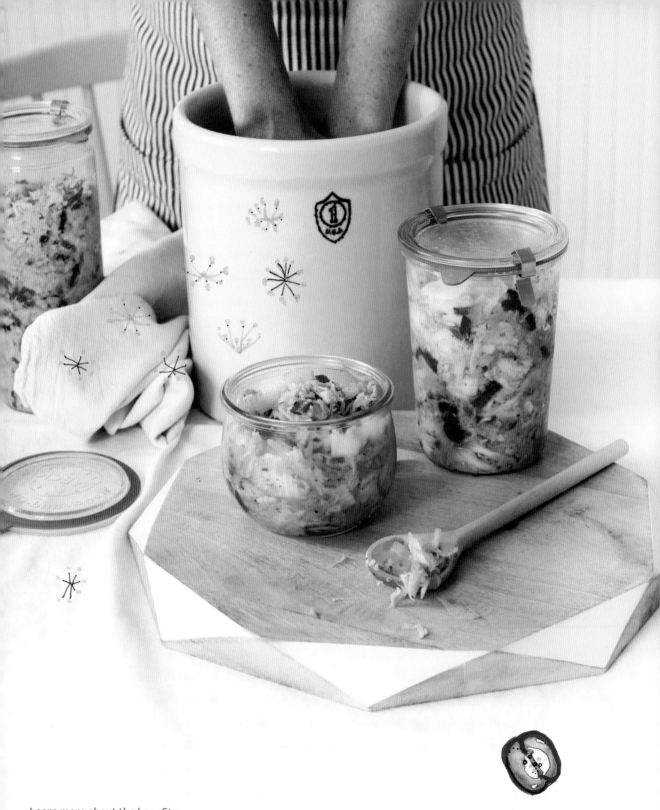

Learn more about the benefits,
safety, and possibilities of fermented foods:
yumuniverse.com/?s=fermented

Fermented Veggies

Long before food manufacturers started making fermented foods like bread, cheese, chocolate, pickles, wine, tea, salami, vinegar, and kombucha, these goods were made at home for thousands of years, all over the world. Instinctually, folks understood that these foods promoted vibrant health, and bonus: It practically makes itself!

In total, we have more microscopic organisms in and on our bodies than we have cells. And fermented foods keep us strong by helping our bodies maintain an important balance so the good guys can flourish. Fermentation makes foods more nutritious, delicious, and shelf stable—it's Mother Nature's preservation technique, and it couldn't be easier or offer up more freestyle variations to play with.

Fermented Veggie combos shown here left to right:
Savoy Cabbage, Kale & Green Apple Kraut (page 156); Fire Breathin'
Fermented Veggies (page 157).

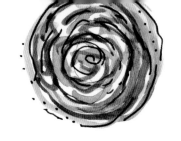

Fermented Veggies

2+ SERVINGS
PREP TIME: 10 TO 15 MINUTES
FERMENTATION TIME: 3 TO 5 DAYS, OR LONGER

Cabbage + salt + time is all you really need to create one of my favorite gateway fermented foods—sauerkraut. This template proposes variations for creating a traditional kraut, but the goal is the same: to get you started (and hooked) on the infinite possibilities for fermented foods because you . . . Can. Do. This.

You'll need 3 to 4 large glass canning jars with a lids, one large 1-gallon (3.8 L) ceramic crock or similar glass vessel (metal and plastic interfere with the fermentation process); a large glass mixing bowl; a grater, food processor, and/or knife; a dish towel; a rubber band; and counter space.

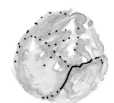

Making kraut doesn't really require exact measurements, but I'm including them here to get you comfy with ratios that work well.

What you need no matter what:

1 to 2 teaspoons sea salt, or more to taste

1 Place Crunch and Main Veg in a large bowl. Prepping in bite-sized pieces creates mucho surface area for bacteria to munch on and in turn ferment. No grater or food processor? Use elbow grease and a knife to prepare tiny pieces.

Crunch ----------- *and* -----------> Main Veg

1 HEAD (3 POUNDS/1.3 KG) TOTAL, CHOPPED, GRATED, OR SLICED
Choose one or combine

Savoy cabbage   Red cabbage

Napa cabbage   Heirloom cabbage

½ TO 2 CUPS CHOPPED, GRATED, OR SLICED TOTAL
Choose one or combine

Carrots (any kind)   Kale (any kind)

Radishes (any kind)   Kohlrabi

Turnips

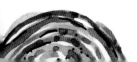

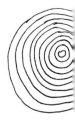

2 Transfer Extras (if using) to the bowl and sprinkle the **salt** evenly over everything and toss. Then taste—it should be very salty, but not overbearing. Squeeze, press, and massage veggies for 7 to 10 minutes, until they break down, wilt, and release water (this is brine). Lift out a handful of veg and squeeze—it should release water like wringing out a wet dish towel. Fold in Flavor (if using) and give a few more squeezes to incorporate the salty brine.

Extras

¼ TO 2 CUPS CORED, SEEDED, SHREDDED/CHOPPED TOTAL
Choose one or combine, or skip altogether

Apples (any kind)

1 to 2 chile peppers

Beets (any kind)

Onion (any kind)

Shallot

Brussels sprouts

Bok choy

Celery

Parsnips

Bell peppers (any kind)

Fennel bulb

Leeks

Flavor

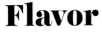

Choose one or combine, or skip altogether

¼ to 1 teaspoon coriander seeds

¼ to 1 teaspoon cumin seeds

¼ to 1 teaspoon mustard seeds

¼ to 1 cinnamon stick

¼ to 1 teaspoon fennel seeds

1 to 2 cardamom pods

5 to 6 garlic cloves, minced

¼ to 1 teaspoon caraway seeds

1 to 3 teaspoons red pepper flakes

¼ to 1 teaspoon dill seeds

1 to 3 tablespoons fresh herbs (thyme, dill, chives, oregano, basil, parsley, cilantro)

¼ to 1 teaspoon peppercorns (white, pink, black, Sichuan)

1 to 2 teaspoons grated turmeric root

1 to 2 teaspoons peeled, grated fresh ginger

¼ to 1 teaspoon juniper berries

1 to 6 teaspoons dried seaweed (dulse, arame, wakame, kombu)

1 to 2 teaspoons grated citrus zest

3 Transfer all the veggies and brine to a large crock or jar—tightly pack down the veggies until submerged under the brine. Put a clean glass plate directly on the veg and something heavy on top of that to weigh it down. The veg has to stay under the salty brine to ferment and protect from mold—the weighted plate makes it so. Cover with a dish towel and secure with a rubber band. Leave on a sun-free part of the counter at room temperature. Ferment for 3 to 5 days, or up to a few weeks (more sour/funky). Sample each day to decide what tastes best. After the fermentation time has passed, you can add some heat and spice before canning. Fold Kick into your fermented veg and repack so it's submerged entirely in brine. Then tightly pack the veggies into canning jars with ¼ inch (6 mm) of brine on top, secure with a lid, and refrigerate. Enjoy right away or within a few months.

Kick

Choose one or combine, or skip altogether

¼ teaspoon chipotle powder

1 to 3 tablespoons harissa (jar), Sriracha, or other hot sauce

¼ to 1 teaspoon chili powder

Old Bay Seasoning

Chinese five-spice

Savoy Cabbage, Kale & Green Apple Kraut

Tart, slightly sweet green apple and cabbage is infused with fragrant juniper berries, caraway, and dill for a kraut that's fantastic on a smoky Veggie Burger (page 235) or swirled into a warm lentil Soup (page 175).

SERVES 8+

1 head green cabbage (3 pounds/1.3 kg), shredded

1 cup (125 g) cored, shredded Granny Smith apple

1 cup (110 g) shredded carrots

1 cup (15 g) stemmed, shredded kale

1 to 2 teaspoons sea salt

½ cup (50 g) chopped celery

½ cup (80 g) diced shallot

3 tablespoons fresh dill

2 teaspoons juniper berries

½ teaspoon caraway seeds

1. Combine the cabbage, apple, carrots, and kale in a large bowl. Sprinkle everything evenly with 1 teaspoon of the salt. Squeeze, press, and massage the veggies for 7 to 10 minutes, until they break down, wilt, and release water (this is brine). Taste the mixture; it should be pretty salty, but not overbearing or inedible at all. Lift out a handful of veg and squeeze— it should release water like wringing out a wet dish towel.

2. Fold in the remaining ingredients and squeeze to incorporate the salty brine. Use your hands to tightly pack down the veggies in a large crock or jar until submerged under the brine. Put a glass plate on the veg and something heavy on top of that to weigh it down. The veg has to stay under brine to ferment. Cover with a dish towel, secure with a rubber band, and leave on a sun-free part of the counter at room temperature for 3 days. Taste on day 3; if you want it to be more sour, let it ferment longer, up to a few weeks. When it tastes good to you, tightly pack into mason jars with ¼ inch (6 mm) of brine on top, secure with a lid, and refrigerate until ready to eat. Kraut keeps for months and months in the fridge.

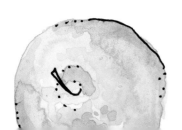

Fire-Breathin' Fermented Veggies

Heat lovers, prepare for addiction. These ingredients
are what you'd use for Korean kimchi, but the
prep here differs a bit from the traditional steps.

SERVES 8+

1 head Napa cabbage
(3 pounds/1.3 kg)

½ cup (75 g) chopped
red bell pepper

½ cup (50 g) chopped scallions

½ cup (60 g) peeled, shredded
daikon radish

½ cup (55 g) shredded carrots

¼ cup (40 g) chopped
yellow onion

6 garlic cloves, diced

1 chile pepper, seeded,
stemmed, and chopped

2 teaspoons sea salt

2 teaspoons peeled, grated
fresh ginger

1 teaspoon dulse flakes

1 teaspoon red pepper flakes

1 to 3 tablespoons Sriracha or
similar-style hot sauce

1   Use a chef's knife to chop the cabbage into bite-sized pieces and transfer to a
bowl with the bell pepper, scallions, daikon, carrots, onion, garlic, and chile.

2   Sprinkle the salt evenly over all. Squeeze, press, and massage the veggies for
7 to 10 minutes, until they break down, wilt, and release water (this is brine).
Taste the mixture; it should be pretty salty, but not overbearing or inedible
at all. Lift out a handful of the veg and squeeze—it should release water like
wringing out a wet dish towel. Fold in the ginger, dulse, and red pepper
flakes and give a few more squeezes to incorporate the salty brine.

3   Use your hands to tightly pack down the veggies into a large crock or jar
until submerged under the brine. Put a glass plate on the veg and something
heavy on top of that to weigh it down. The veg has to stay under brine to
ferment. Cover with a dish towel, secure with a rubber band, and leave
on a sun-free part of the counter at room temperature for at least 3 days.
Taste on day 3; if you want it to be more sour, let it ferment longer, up to a
few weeks. When it tastes good to you, drain the brine, toss the veggies with
1 tablespoon Sriracha and taste. Add more Sriracha until it satisfies your
heat requirements. Tightly pack the mixture into mason jars with ¼ inch
(6 mm) of brine on top, secure with a lid, and refrigerate until ready to eat.
Fermented Veggies keep for months and months in the fridge.

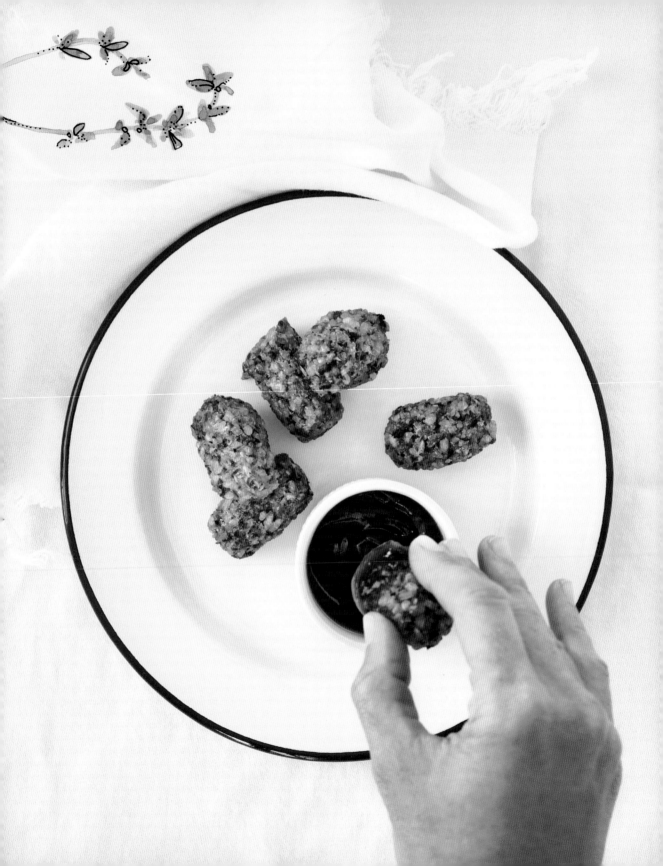

Bites & Tots

This is the stuff of childhood memories, bite-sized goodness only better! We're taking this classic finger food to the next level with more flavor, color, texture, and nutrients.

Bites and tots make meal- and snack-time easier. Simply prepare a few batches, freeze, and bake up later, or go ahead and bake them up, store in the fridge for a few weeks, and reheat in the oven when hungry.

Serve them as appetizers for entertaining and don't forget: They're simply the perfect vehicle for amazing sauces of all kinds, so check out page 28 for inspiration to dress each bite.

Tots combo shown here:
Sweet potato, cauliflower, brown rice & thyme.

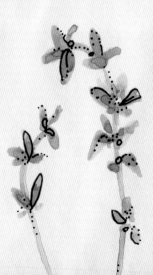

Bites & Tots

MAKES 24 TO 36
COOK TIME: 15 TO 20 MINUTES

You'll need a food processor for this recipe, but in a pinch, good old-fashioned elbow grease and a masher or fork can work. I call for psyllium husk as the binder because it's hands-down the strongest. I bet you can use an egg if you eat them. This template calls for baking the tots, but you can also pan fry them in a greased skillet heated to medium-high—use tongs to turn tots so they brown a few minutes on each side.

Volume and quantity of individual ingredients, how they react to sautéing, and the size you ultimately shape your bites and tots will create differences in the yield—halve, double, or triple batches if you need to and use the following recipes as a gauge for what to expect.

What you need no matter what:

2 to 3 teaspoons unrefined coconut oil or grapeseed oil

½ cup (80 g) diced onion (any kind) or shallot

1 to 3 garlic cloves, minced (optional)

1¼ teaspoons ground psyllium husk

¼ teaspoon sea salt,
plus more to taste

1 Preheat the oven to 400°F (200°C)—line a baking sheet with unbleached parchment paper. In a skillet heated to medium, add the **oil** and sauté Base, Veggies, and **onion** for 7 minutes, or until softened. Add the **garlic** (if using) and sauté for 2 to 3 more minutes.

Base ------- *and* -------→ Veggies

½ CUP SHREDDED/GRATED TOTAL
Choose one or combine

Sweet potatoes	Beets
Winter squash	Potatoes (any kind)
	Carrots

½ CUP CHOPPED TOTAL
Choose one or combine

Bell pepper (any kind)	Green peas
Celery	Mushrooms
Broccoli	Summer squash
Cauliflower	Hearty greens

2 Transfer the cooked veggies to the food processor and evenly sprinkle the **psyllium** around everything. Add Texture, Protein (if using), and the **salt**—pulse 5 to 10 times to break apart. Season with more salt if needed.

Texture ⸺ *and/or* ⸺→ Protein

1 CUP COOKED
Choose one or combine;
page 11 for cooking tips

Buckwheat, hulled

Short-grain
brown rice

½ CUP COOKED TOTAL
Choose one or combine, or skip
altogether; page 11 for cooking tips

Beans (any kind)

Chickpeas

Lentils

3 Add Flavor (if using) to the food processor and pulse 5 to 20 more times until the mixture breaks up and starts to stick together, but don't overprocess into a paste; you want to maintain texture and color. Add more Flavor if you like.

Flavor

Choose one or combine, or skip altogether

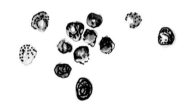

1 tablespoon to ¼ cup (10 g) fresh herbs	1 to 3 teaspoons fresh citrus juice	Fresh-cracked black pepper
½ to 1 teaspoon grated citrus zest	1 to 2 teaspoons nutritional yeast	1 to 4 teaspoons of your favorite seasoning mix

4 Take a small cereal-spoonful of mixture from the food processor and lightly squeeze it in your palm so it sticks together—use your other hand to shape it into a tot (cylinder) or bite (round) in your palm; place on the lined baking sheet. Repeat until all the mixture is used up. Some mixtures are stickier than others; washing your hands a few times between rolling helps! Bake for 15 to 20 minutes, until the outside is browned and crispy. Enjoy with dipping sauce (see pages 28 to 33).

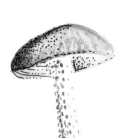

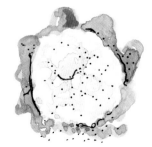

Buckwheat & Chickpea Bites

If you or any kiddos in your life like chicken tenders,
these are a tasty plant-packed option to try.
Great dipped in a ranch dressing, Chipotle Cream
(page 28), or Smoky BBQ Sauce (page 30).

MAKES 24 TO 36

1 tablespoon unrefined coconut or grapeseed oil

½ cup (80 g) diced yellow onion

½ cup (70 g) peeled, seeded, and shredded acorn squash

½ cup (8 g) shredded kale (any kind)

2 garlic cloves, minced

1 cup (170 g) cooked hulled buckwheat groats (roughly ½ cup/80 g dry; see page 11)

½ cup (80 g) cooked chickpeas (roughly ¼ cup/50 g dry; see page 11)

1¼ teaspoons ground psyllium husk

¼ teaspoon sea salt, plus more to taste

2 teaspoons fresh lemon juice

1 teaspoon fresh parsley

1 teaspoon fresh sage leaves

1 teaspoon fresh thyme

Fresh-cracked black pepper

Smoky BBQ Sauce (page 30) or store-bought

1. Preheat the oven to 400°F (200°C) and line a baking sheet with unbleached parchment paper.

2. In a skillet heated to medium, add the oil and sauté the onion, squash, and kale for 7 minutes, or until softened and browning. Add the garlic and sauté for 3 more minutes.

3. Transfer the veggies to a food processor and evenly sprinkle the psyllium around everything. Add the buckwheat, chickpeas, and salt—pulse 20 times to break apart. Season with more salt to taste.

4. Add the lemon juice, parsley, sage, thyme, and a few grinds of pepper to the food processor and pulse 10 to 20 more times, until the mixture breaks up and starts to stick together—don't overprocess into a paste; you want to maintain texture and color. Take a small spoonful of the mixture and lightly squeeze it in your palm so it sticks together—use your other hand to shape it into a bite-sized mini-burger patty and place on the lined baking sheet. Repeat until all the mixture is used up. Bake for 15 minutes, or until browned and crispy—enjoy warm with BBQ Sauce.

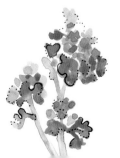

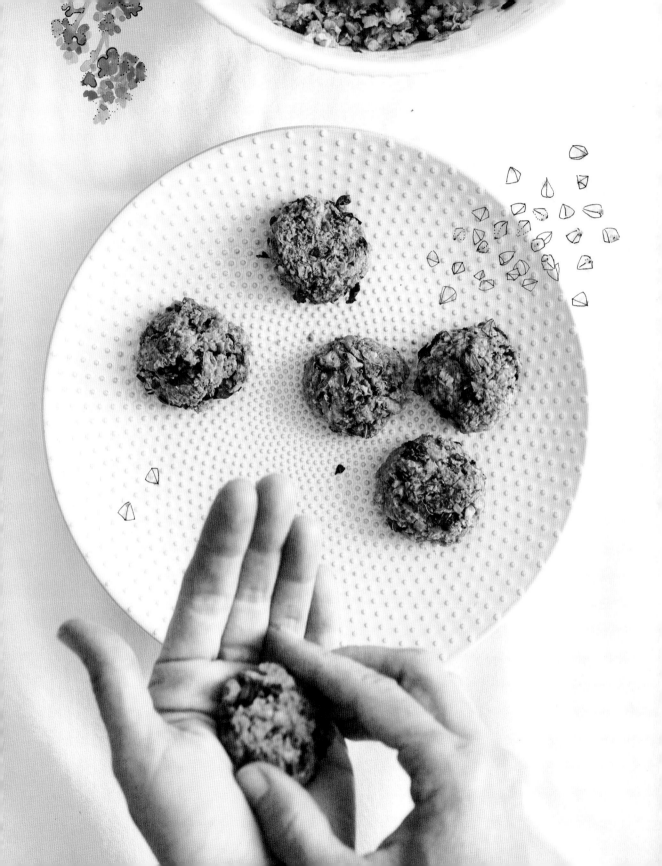

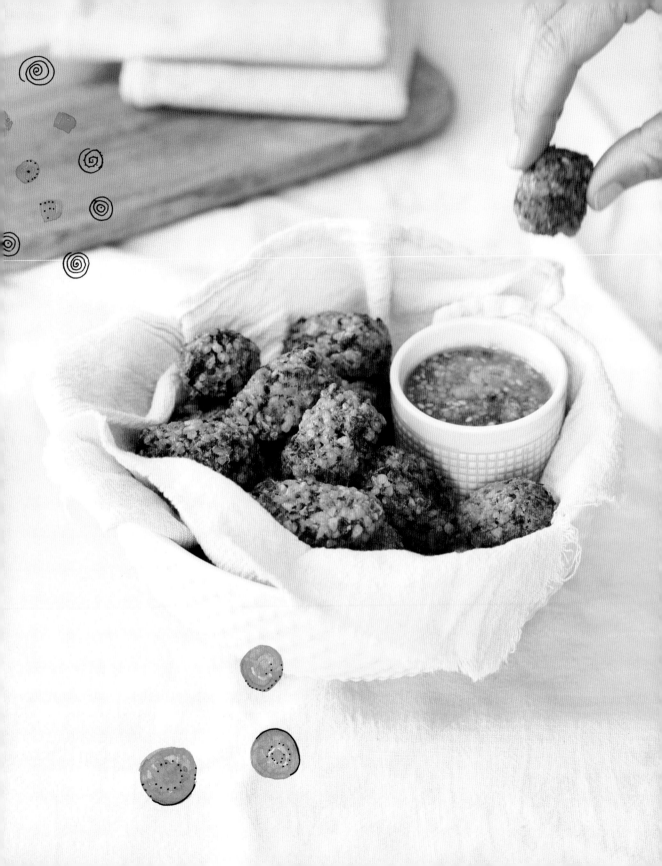

Carrot & Cauliflower Tots *with* Orange-Sesame Dipping Sauce

Savory tots with a sweet, citrusy dipping sauce. If you're crunched for time, buy an organic Asian-style sauce you like for dipping instead of making homemade.

MAKES 24 TO 36

Orange-Sesame Sauce (page 30)

1 tablespoon unrefined coconut or grapeseed oil

½ cup (50 g) chopped cauliflower florets

½ cup (80 g) diced white onion

½ cup (55 g) shredded carrots

1¼ teaspoons ground psyllium husk

1 cup (195 g) cooked short-grain brown rice (roughly ½ cup/90 g dry; page 11 for tips)

¼ teaspoon sea salt, plus more to taste

2 tablespoons fresh cilantro

1 teaspoon fresh lime juice

½ teaspoon grated lime zest (optional)

1. Preheat the oven to 400°F (200°C) and line a baking sheet with unbleached parchment paper or a silicone baking mat. Then run the Orange-Sesame Sauce through a food processor or blender until smooth and positively dippable—set aside.

2. In a skillet heated to medium, add the oil and sauté the carrots, onion, and cauliflower for 7 minutes, or until softened. Transfer the contents of skillet to the food processor, and evenly sprinkle the psyllium around everything. Add the rice and salt and pulse 15 to 20 times to roughly incorporate. Season with more salt if you like.

3. Add the cilantro, lime juice, and lime zest (if using) to the food processor and pulse 20 to 25 more times. Don't overprocess; you want to maintain texture and color, but break up the ingredients enough that they just begin to clump together. Take a small cereal-spoonful of the mixture from the food processor and lightly squeeze it in your palm so it sticks together— use your other hand to shape it into a tot in your palm; place on the lined baking sheet. Repeat until all the mixture is used up. Bake for 20 minutes, or until browned and crispy. Enjoy warm plunged into Orange-Sesame Dipping Sauce.

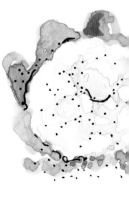

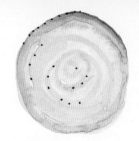

Veggie Fries

Let's go beyond the white potato and bring more nutrition, color, and flavor to our fries with a variety of veggies. Final fry texture varies with these baked options, from crispy outside with a firm interior (hi, yuca) to caramelized exterior with a surprising, watery pop inside (hello, radish).

Load them with vibrant seasoning before baking or keep it simple with a little S&P. Make a creamy, cooling Dip (page 137) or sauce (page 28) to enjoy them with.

Run firm veggies through a spiralizer for curly fries, or cut them into skinny matchsticks or big, fat wedges.

Want to make mixed veggie fries? Choose ingredients with similar bake times, or add quicker-cooking ingredients after longer-cooking ingredients have baked the difference in times already. Remember, the thicker the fry, the longer it takes to cook, so adjust.

Veggie Fries shown here:
Red beet, sweet potato, golden beet, carrot, yuca.

4+ SERVINGS
PREP TIME: 5 TO 15 MINUTES

What you need no matter what:

¼ teaspoon sea salt, plus more to taste

 1 Preheat the oven to 425°F (220°C) and line a baking sheet with unbleached parchment paper. If using jicama, winter squash, or yuca, remove the skin. You can peel the other Veggies, but it's not necessary. Remove the seeds from winter squash.

Veggies

3 CUPS STRIPS OR WEDGES TOTAL
Choose one or combine; note bake times and adjust if they differ.

Beets
Bake: 20 to 30 minutes

Carrots
Bake: 20 to 30 minutes

Daikon radish
Bake: 20 to 30 minutes

Green beans
Bake: 10 to 15 minutes

Jicama
Bake: 10 to 15 minutes

Parsnip
Bake: 15 to 20 minutes

Purple potatoes
Bake: 30 to 35 minutes

Rutabaga
Bake: 20 to 30 minutes

Sweet potatoes
Bake: 20 to 25 minutes

Turnips
Bake: 20 to 30 minutes

Winter squash (delicata, kabocha, acorn, butternut, pumpkin)
Bake: 20 to 30 minutes

Yuca (a.k.a. cassava)
Bake: 20 to 30 minutes

 2 In a bowl, toss Veggies with the **salt** (skip this salt if using a salted seasoning mix for Flavor like Old Bay) and Oil until evenly coated. Spread onto the baking sheet so the fries have room to brown on all sides. Bake for half of the time specified above, remove from the oven, and stir in Flavor and Crunch (if using). Also stir in 1 to 4 minced garlic cloves at this point if you like; finish baking until crispy and brown. Season with more salt to taste.

Oil

2 TO 4 TABLESPOONS TOTAL
Choose one

Unrefined coconut oil, gently warmed to liquid

Grapeseed oil

Avocado oil

Flavor

Choose any in combination, or skip altogether

1 to 3 teaspoons nutritional yeast

¼ to ½ teaspoon chipotle powder

2 to 4 tablespoons harissa (jar)

2 to 4 tablespoons Dijon or whole-grain mustard

1 to 3 tablespoons vinegar (any kind)

1 to 2 tablespoons Old Bay

½ to 1 teaspoon garam masala

½ to 1 teaspoon ground cumin

¼ teaspoon cayenne pepper

¼ to ½ teaspoons grated citrus zest

1 to 4 teaspoons chopped fresh herbs (rosemary, thyme, sage, dill, chives, oregano, basil, parsley, cilantro)

1 to 3 teaspoons miso

1 to 3 teaspoons Sriracha

2 to 4 tablespoons za'atar spice blend

½ to 2 teaspoons paprika (smoked or plain)

1 to 2 tablespoons maple syrup

Crunch

2 TO 3 TABLESPOONS
Choose one, mix, or skip altogether

Seeds, chopped into small pieces (sunflower, pepitas)

Almond flour

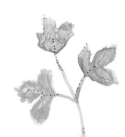

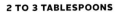

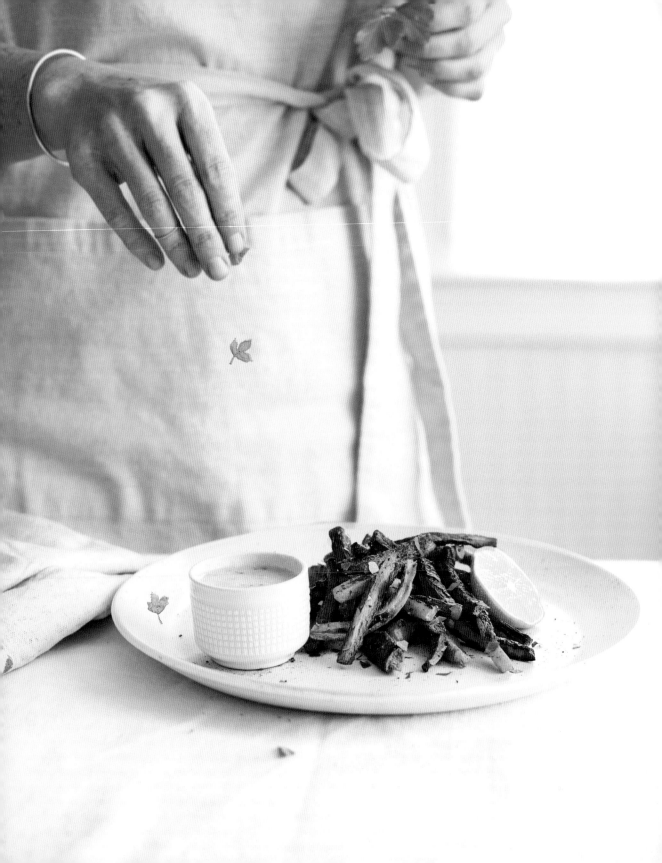

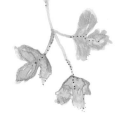

Chesapeake Carrot Fries

As a Maryland gal, I'm happy to share with you a
recipe using one of our culinary treasures—Old Bay Seasoning.
It has a spicy tastes-like-summer-by-the-shore flavor that
pairs so well with sweet rainbow carrots (you can use
any kind you find, actually, even non-rainbows). Know that
the Honey Mustard Dipping Sauce also makes a great
salad dressing, so use any extra for an Epic Salad (page 195).

SERVES 4+

Honey Mustard Dipping Sauce
(optional)

¾ cup (105 g) raw, unsalted
cashews, soaked for 4 to 6 hours

¼ cup plus 2 tablespoons (90 ml)
water, plus more if needed

3 tablespoons raw,
unpasteurized honey

3 tablespoons Dijon or
whole-grain mustard

1 tablespoon plus ½ teaspoon
fresh lemon juice

¼ teaspoon sea salt,
or more to taste

Fries

4 to 5 large carrots, sliced
into thin 3- to 4-inch (7.5 to
10 cm) strips (skin on for
extra texture and nutrients,
or peeled if desired)

¼ cup (60 ml) grapeseed oil

Fresh-cracked black pepper

1 to 2 tablespoons
Old Bay, to taste

1 teaspoon fresh parsley

½ teaspoon grated lemon zest

Sea salt

1. Blend together all the Honey Mustard Dipping Sauce ingredients (if using)
   until ultra-smooth. Season with more salt if you like, and add more water,
   1 tablespoon at a time, until you reach the desired consistency for dipping;
   set aside. Preheat the oven to 425°F (220°C) and line a baking sheet with
   unbleached parchment paper.

2. In a large bowl, toss together the carrots and oil until the carrots are
   thoroughly coated. Spread evenly on the baking sheet so each fry has
   room to brown on all sides—no stacking. Grind fresh pepper over all.

3. Bake for 15 minutes. Remove from the oven and sprinkle the Old Bay,
   parsley, and lemon zest all over the fries—give them a stir and spread
   them back out on the sheet. Return to the oven and bake for another 5 to
   15 minutes, until crispy and brown. Season with salt to taste if you like.
   Allow to cool a bit, but serve warm with the Honey Mustard Dipping Sauce.

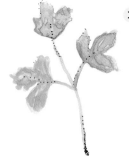

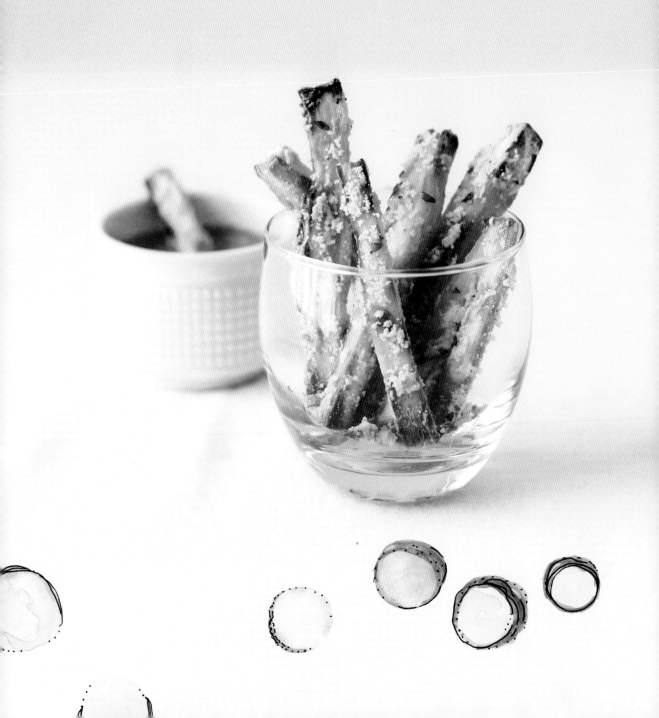

Cheesy Yuca Fries

Crunchy, cheesy flavor created from nutritious
nuts and seeds covers firm yet tender yuca root—
these are fries, elevated.

SERVES 4+

½ cup (55 g) blanched
almond flour

¼ cup (35 g) raw,
unsalted cashews

¼ cup (35 g) raw, unsalted
pine nuts

2 tablespoons
nutritional yeast

¾ teaspoon sea salt,
plus more to taste

1 to 2 large yucas, peeled and
sliced into thin 3- to 4-inch
(7.5 to 10 cm) strips
(about 3 cups/600 g)

1 teaspoon fresh parsley

3 tablespoons unrefined
coconut oil

1 tablespoon apple cider vinegar

Chimichurri
(optional, page 30), blended

1. Preheat the oven to 425°F (220°C) and line a baking sheet with unbleached
   parchment paper.

2. In a food processor or coffee or spice grinder, pulse together the flour,
   cashews, and pine nuts until pulverized, but not a paste. Transfer to a small
   bowl and fold together with the nutritional yeast and ½ teaspoon of the
   salt. It should be a bit sticky and clumpy, like feta or goat cheese. Set aside.

3. In a large bowl, toss together the yuca, oil, vinegar, and remaining ¼ teaspoon
   salt until thoroughly coated. Spread evenly on the baking sheet so each fry
   has room to brown on all sides—no stacking. Bake for 15 minutes. Remove
   from the oven and sprinkle the cheesy mixture over the fries—press the
   cheese onto the fries a bit and then spread back out on the sheet. Return to
   the oven and bake for another 5 to 10 minutes, until crispy and brown.
   Season with more salt if needed. Allow to cool a bit, but serve warm with
   the Chimichurri.

Seed-Powered Acorn Squash Fries

A simple combo of garlic, salt, and pepper on any veggies fries
is all you really need for a tasty fry fix. But why stop there?
Add toasty crunch from pepitas and sunflower seeds and pair
with addictive Chipotle Cream. You're welcome.
And leftover dipping sauce can be used for a Massaged
Kale & Mango Salad (page 198).

SERVES 4+

2 medium acorn squash

¼ cup (60 ml) unrefined
coconut oil, gently warmed
to liquid

½ teaspoon sea salt

¼ cup (30 g) raw, unsalted
pepitas, chopped into
small pieces

¼ cup (35 g) raw, unsalted
sunflower seeds, chopped
into small pieces

3 to 4 garlic cloves, minced

1 teaspoon paprika (smoked
or plain—chef's choice)

Chipotle Cream
(optional: page 28)

1. Preheat the oven to 425°F (220°C) and line a baking sheet with unbleached
parchment paper. Remove the skin and seeds from the squash, slice the
squash from top to bottom into ¼-inch (6 mm) thick slices—then slice those
squash slices into fries. You will end up with a few non-fry-like strips—
keep them to cook up, too.

2. In a large bowl, toss together the squash, oil, and salt until thoroughly
coated. Taste and season with more salt if you think it's necessary. Spread
evenly on the baking sheet so each fry has room to brown on all sides—
no stacking. Bake for 15 minutes. Remove from the oven and sprinkle the
pepitas, sunflower seeds, garlic, and paprika all over the fries—give them
a stir to mix everything together well and spread back out on the sheet.
Return to the oven and bake for another 5 to 15 minutes, until crispy and
brown. Allow to cool a bit, but serve warm with Chipotle Cream.

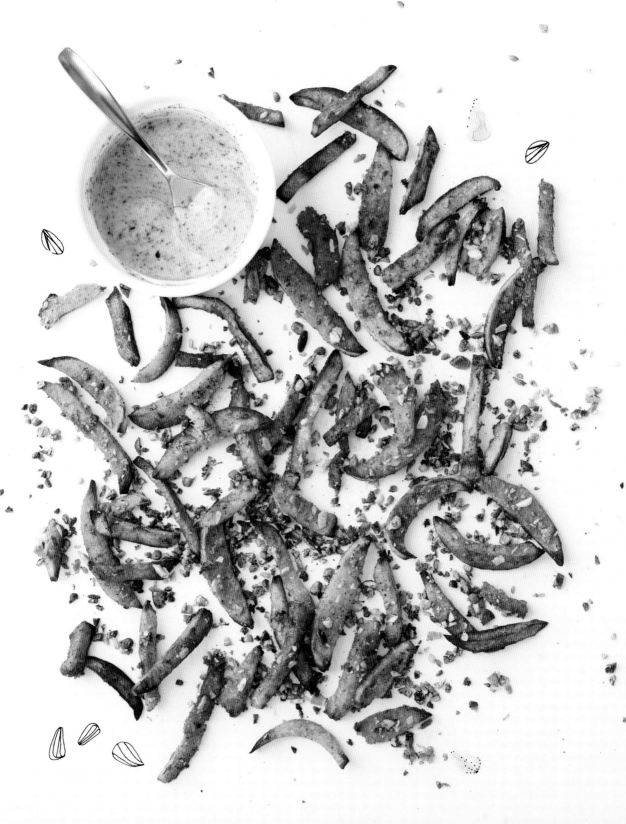

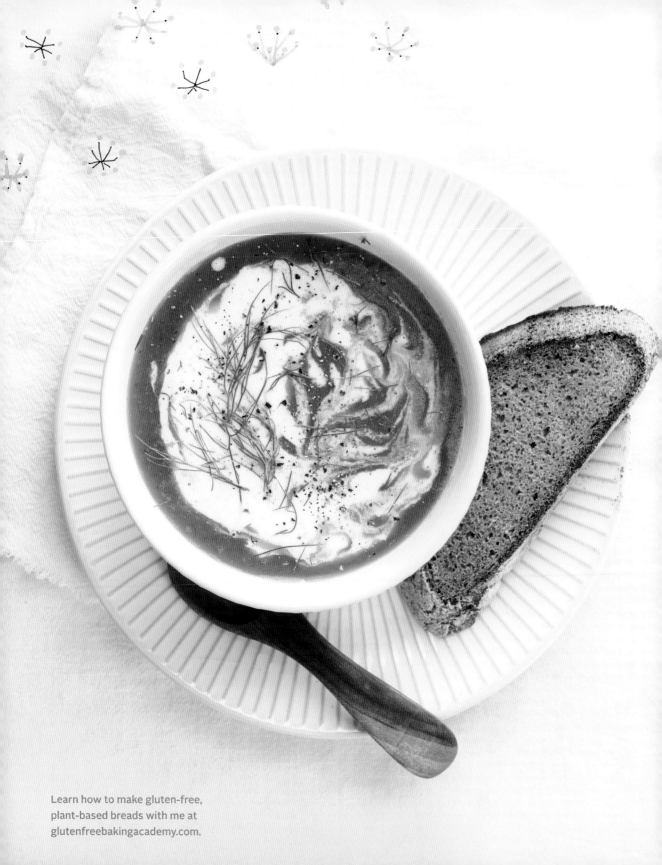

Learn how to make gluten-free,
plant-based breads with me at
glutenfreebakingacademy.com.

Soups

If you start with simple aromatics (page 20 for tips),
add some veggie stock, and maybe some texture
from fruit, veggies, grains, and/or beans, you can have
a comforting bowl of soup in minutes.

It's the ultimate freestyle since you can use what
you have, right now, in your kitchen. Even if you don't
have any veggie stock on hand, you can make
some by boiling water, veggies scraps, an onion,
maybe some garlic and herbs—strain, done.

So, save those cooking veggie scraps throughout the
week (freezer or fridge) to use for stock. And then freeze
homemade stock in ice cube trays and jars for
months of quick soup making, grain cooking, sautéing,
and other pantry-to-plate freestyles.

Soup combo shown here:
Pumpkin, garlic, dill, nutmeg & coconut cream.

Soups

4 TO 6 SERVINGS
COOK TIME: 30 TO 45 MINUTES

Try a simple stock filled with vegetables, and maybe add some noodles or rice. Always start with less water or broth and add more until you reach the desired consistency. Blend half of a batch of soup and add the purée back into the pot to thicken and add "bulk" to a soup, or you can purée it all for decadent, smooth spoonful after spoonful. If you can imagine it, you can make it—just be sure to choose ingredients you *like* to eat.

What you need no matter what

1 to 2 tablespoons coconut or grapeseed oil

1 to 6 garlic cloves (optional), minced

4 to 6 cups (1 to 1.4 L) low-sodium veggie stock or water

1 teaspoon sea salt, or more to taste

1 In a large soup pot heated to medium, add the **oil** and sauté diced Dense Veggies (if using) for 10 to 20 minutes, until easily pierced with a fork, but firm and not mushy.

Dense Veggies

1 TO 3 CUPS DICED TOTAL
Choose one or combine, or skip altogether

Sweet potatoes	Beets
Winter squash, peeled and seeded	Potatoes (any kind)

2 Add sliced or diced Aromatics to the pot. Sauté over medium heat for 7 to 10 minutes until veggies are "sweating" and starting to brown.

Aromatics

Choose one or combine, sliced or diced

1 to 2 onions (any)	1 to 3 large carrots	2 to 10 scallions
1 to 2 shallots	1 to 3 celery stalks	1 tablespoon to ¼ cup (10 g) fresh herbs (dill, basil, sage, rosemary, parsley, marjoram, cilantro, oregano, chives)
1 to 2 bell peppers	1 to 5 leeks, white and light green parts only	
1- to 2-inch (5 cm) piece fresh ginger, peeled and grated	1 to 2 chile peppers, seeded	

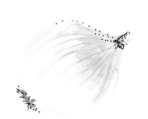

3 Add sliced or diced Fruit & Veg to the pot. Sauté over medium heat for 5 to 7 minutes until softening. If you want, add the **garlic,** stirring for an additional 2 to 3 minutes. Add Flavor (if using)—stir for 1 minute, then add the **stock;** bring to a boil.

Fruit & Veg ----- *and/or* -----→ Flavor

1 TO 4 CUPS SLICED OR DICED TOTAL
Choose one or combine

Choose one or combine, or skip altogether

Pome fruit (any kind), cored

Tomatoes

Hearty greens (kale, chard, spinach)

Summer squash

Turnips

Celeriac

Mushrooms

Cabbage

Carrots

Bell peppers (any)

Celery

Cauliflower

Broccoli

Fennel bulb

Asparagus

Green peas/ sugar snap peas

¼ to ½ teaspoon liquid smoke

1 to 3 teaspoons paprika (smoked or plain)

1 to 3 teaspoons ground cumin

1 to 3 teaspoons chipotle powder

¼ to 1 teaspoon ground cinnamon

Pinch to ¼ teaspoon fresh-ground nutmeg

1 to 3 teaspoons ground coriander

1 bay leaf

Pinch to ¼ teaspoon ground cardamom

1 to 3 tablespoons curry paste (any)

¼ to ½ cup (60 to 120 ml) dry red or white wine

½ to 2 teaspoons vinegar (red wine, white wine, rice wine, apple cider, sherry)

½ to 3 teaspoons fresh citrus juice

¼ to 1 teaspoon grated citrus zest

1 to 3 teaspoons ground turmeric

¼ to 3 cups (60 to 720 ml) canned coconut milk

¼ to 1 cup (60 to 240 ml) Cashew Cream (page 32)

4 Reduce the heat to a simmer; cook for 5 minutes. Fold in Texture (if using); cook for another 5 to 10 minutes. Stir in the **salt,** spoon into a serving bowl, and add Finishing Touches (if using).

Texture

1 TO 4 CUPS SLICED OR DICED TOTAL
Choose one or combine, or skip altogether; page 11 for cooking tips

Beans (any kind), cooked

Buckwheat, hulled and cooked

Chickpeas, cooked

Lentils, cooked

Millet, cooked

Quinoa, cooked

Rice (any), cooked

Noodles (any), cooked al dente

Veggie noodles: raw summer squash or carrots peeled into ribbons or spiralized

Finishing Touches

Choose one or combine, or skip altogether

Fresh-cracked black pepper

Cashew Cream (page 32)

Coconut cream (skimmed from a chilled can of coconut milk)

Scallions, sliced

Fresh herbs, chopped

Crunchies (page 145)

Crouton(s)

Fresh lemon juice

Cashew-Almond Cheese Crumbles (page 133)

Avocado

Roasted nut & seed oils

Extra virgin olive oil

Supergreen Pesto (page 33)

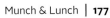

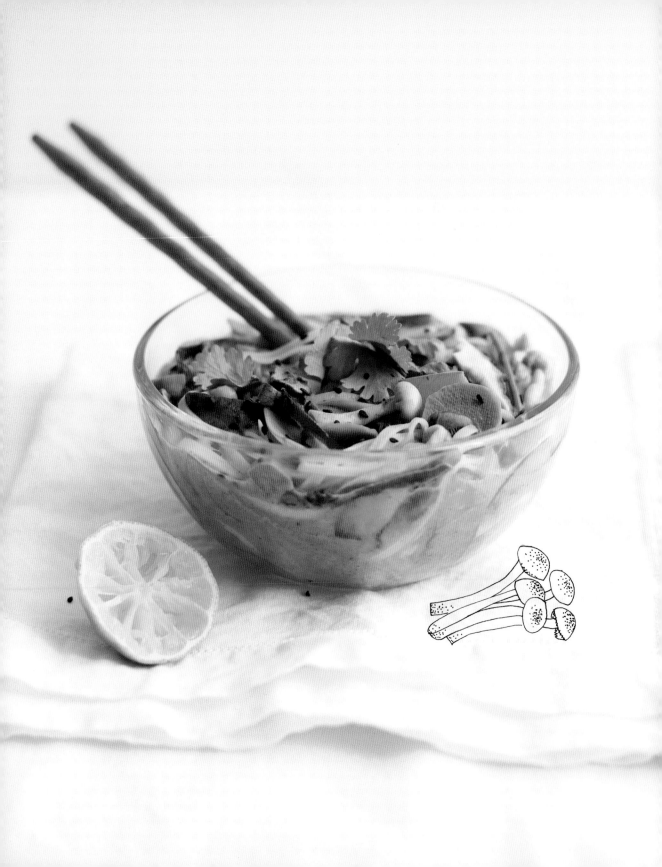

Lots-a-Noodles Red Curry Soup

I make variations of this soup all the time. No tomatoes on hand?
Keep some tomato sauce in the pantry and use that.
Instead of carrots, try sweet winter squash or sweet potatoes.
You can use Italian-style noodles in a pinch—it's all about the broth.
Sometimes, I'll use the whole box of noodles, sometimes
only half. Chef's choice on that one.

SERVES 8+

2 tablespoons unrefined coconut oil

1 red bell pepper, seeded, ribs removed, and sliced

1 large shallot, sliced thinly

1-inch (2.5 cm) piece ginger, peeled and grated—almost a pulp

One 8-ounce (227 g) box gluten-free Asian brown rice noodles

3 cups (210 g) mushrooms (variety: shiitake, beech, button)

1 cup (180 g) diced tomatoes

1 cup (130 g) sliced carrots

1 cup (100 g) sugar snap peas

4 garlic cloves, minced

3 tablespoons red curry paste

2 teaspoons fresh lime juice, plus more for garnish

5 cups (1.2 L) low-sodium vegetable stock

3 cups (720 ml) canned coconut milk

1½ teaspoons sea salt, plus more to taste

Handful fresh cilantro

Toasted sesame seeds (optional)

1. In a large soup pot over medium heat, add the oil and sauté the pepper, shallot, and ginger for 7 to 10 minutes, until soft and starting to brown.

2. Fill another pot with water and bring to a boil. Prepare either the full box (recommended for the "Lots-a-Noodles" aspect) or half box of noodles according to the package instructions.

3. Add the mushrooms, tomatoes, carrots, and snap peas to the pot. Sauté over medium heat for 5 minutes, until the veggies soften a bit. Add the garlic, curry paste, and lime juice—stir for an additional 2 minutes. Add the stock and coconut milk; bring to a boil. Reduce the heat to a simmer, fold in the cooked and drained noodles, and simmer for 5 minutes. Stir in the salt. Serve warm topped with fresh cilantro, a sprinkle of toasted sesame seeds if you like, and a squeeze of fresh lime juice.

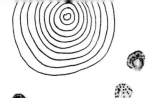

Apple & Onion Soup

Sweet apples and onions combine with floral notes from nutmeg and cardamom for a decadent yet simple soup. For a slightly sour version, try Granny Smith apples instead. Serve it warm with Smoky Coconut Crunch (page 149) or chilled for a changeup.

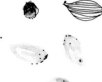

SERVES 4+

One 13.5-ounce (400 ml) can coconut milk

1 tablespoon unrefined coconut oil

1 yellow onion, diced

1-inch (2.5 cm) piece ginger root, peeled and grated—almost a pulp

4 cups (500 g) cored, diced Pink Lady or Honeycrisp apples (2 to 3 apples)

4 cups (960 ml) low-sodium vegetable stock

¼ teaspoon fresh-ground nutmeg

Pinch ground cardamom

1 teaspoon sea salt, or more to taste

—

Topping ideas (optional):

Roasted walnut oil

Fresh-cracked black pepper

1. Whisk together the contents of the can of coconut milk and set aside 1 to 2 tablespoons for garnish—you'll pour the rest into the soup with the stock, so set it aside for now.

2. In a large soup pot over medium heat, add the coconut oil and sauté the onion and ginger for 7 to 10 minutes, until soft and starting to brown.

3. Add the apples to the pot and continue to sauté for 5 to 7 minutes, until softened. Add the stock, coconut milk, nutmeg, and cardamom and bring to a boil. Reduce the heat to a simmer and cook for 7 to 10 minutes.

4. Transfer to a blender to purée until smooth. Stir in the salt. Serve warm and drizzle with the reserved coconut milk and, if you like, the walnut oil and pepper.

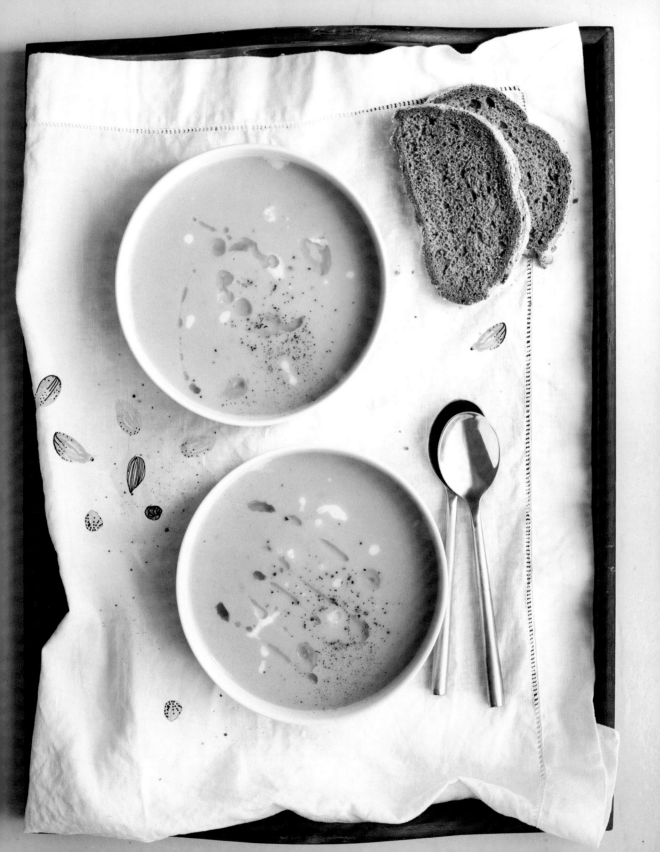

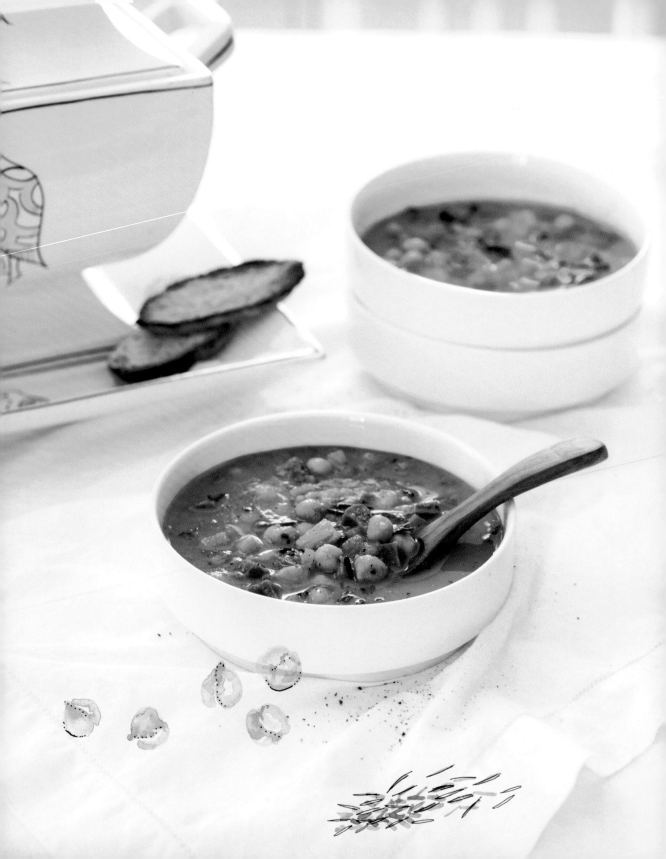

Hearty Chickpea Stew

This is an involved spend-a-Sunday-in-the-kitchen kind of meal—
its hearty, comforting flavor is worth it. To infuse even more
flavor, simmer on low for an additional 20 minutes. Try black quinoa
instead of wild rice for a tasty change and don't forget to dip
in some Crackers from page 112 or a warm savory Muffin (page 63)
spread with coconut oil and a pinch of sea salt.

SERVES 8+

1 tablespoon unrefined
coconut oil

1 yellow onion, diced

3 stalks celery, diced

2 carrots, diced

1 tablespoon fresh thyme

1 cup (15 g) lightly packed
stemmed, chopped kale

¼ cup (60 ml) dry white
wine (optional)

2 teaspoons fresh lemon juice

1 bay leaf

1 teaspoon ground cumin

1 teaspoon ground coriander

½ teaspoon ground turmeric

½ teaspoon smoked paprika

¼ teaspoon grated lemon zest

¼ teaspoon ground cinnamon

5 cups (1.2 L) low-sodium
vegetable stock

3 cups (495 g) cooked chickpeas
(roughly 1 cup/200 g dry;
see page 11)

1 cup (165 g) cooked wild rice,
cooked (roughly ½ cup/80 g dry;
see page 11)

1 teaspoon sea salt, plus
more to taste

Fresh-cracked black pepper

1. Preheat the oven to 425°F (220°C). In a large soup pot or Dutch oven over medium heat, add the oil and sauté the onion, celery, carrots, and thyme for 7 to 10 minutes, until softened and browning.

2. Add the kale; sauté over medium heat for 5 minutes. Add the wine (if using), lemon juice, bay leaf, cumin, coriander, turmeric, paprika, zest, and cinnamon; stir for 2 minutes, then add the stock and bring to a boil. Reduce the heat to a simmer and cook for 5 to 7 minutes.

3. Fold in the chickpeas and wild rice—cook for another 5 minutes. Stir in the salt and then transfer 2 cups (480 ml) of soup (make sure the bay leaf stays in the soup pot and not in the measuring cup) to a blender and purée until smooth. Return the purée to the soup to add bulk, and stir. Reduce the heat to low and season with more salt if you like and generous pepper.

4. Simmer for 10 to 20 minutes to infuse flavor even more—serve warm and enjoy how the flavors develop every day you have any leftovers.

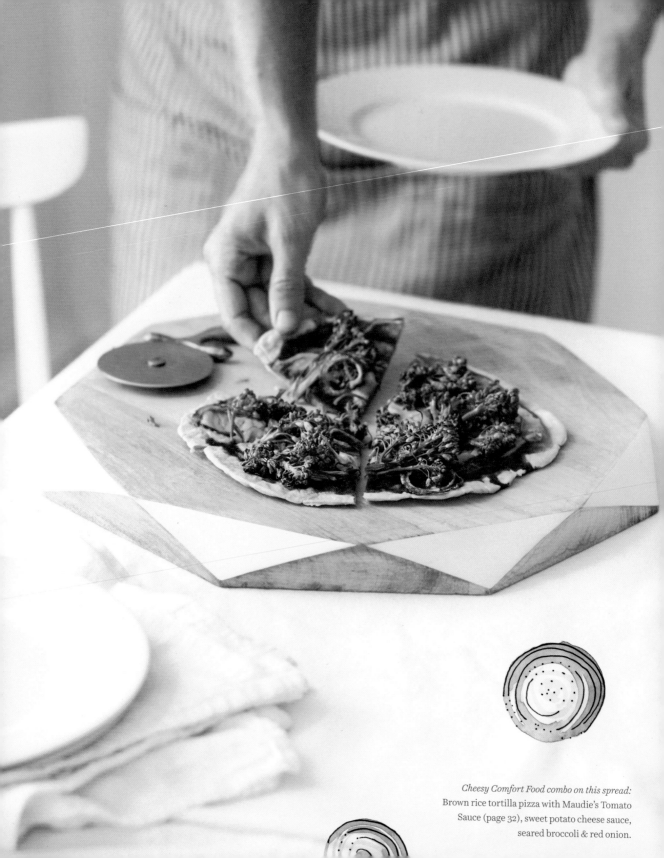

Cheesy Comfort Food combo on this spread:
Brown rice tortilla pizza with Maudie's Tomato
Sauce (page 32), sweet potato cheese sauce,
seared broccoli & red onion.

Main Meals

I'M NOT CALLING THIS SECTION "DINNER," because some folks eat their main meals of the day for lunch or breakfast. Sometimes, a main meal in the evening can be a ginormous mixing-bowl salad loaded with so much color and goodness that it qualifies as a proper "dinner." Make your own rules, but know that the following pages bring vegetables from side dish to superstar center-plate status. Veggie burgers and sliders, lasagna, sushi, creamy macaroni, and tacos never tasted so good.

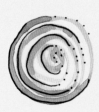

Cheesy Comfort Food

COOK TIME: 15 TO 35 MINUTES

A puréed combination of certain vegetables with a little acid, a little salt, and maybe a little cream makes some of the richest, cheesiest, most decadent dairy-free sauces that any milk "lover" or "avoider" ever had.

This template is all about the sauce, which can transform vegetables, noodles, rice, grains, or legumes into guilt-free comfort food in a matter of minutes. Onion and/or garlic add depth, while acid and nutty-tasting ingredients like nutritional yeast or pine nuts are key for adding cheese-flavored "funk."

A note about soaking cashews and sunflower seeds: It's recommended for nutritional benefit, plus waterlogging them makes for extra-creamy sauces—which is helpful if you don't have a high-powered blender. Skip the soaking step if you're in a pinch—just blend a loooong time.

What you need no matter what:

½ cup (120 ml) water, or more if needed

2 teaspoons unrefined coconut oil or grapeseed oil (optional)

1 teaspoon sea salt, or more to taste

Fresh-cracked black pepper to taste (optional)

1 Roast or steam Veggies (if using) until they're easily pierced with a fork yet firm, not mushy. Transfer to a blender.

Veggies

2 CUPS PEELED AND DICED TOTAL
Choose one or skip altogether

Sweet potatoes	Kabocha squash	Hubbard squash
Buttercup squash	Carnival squash	Red kuri squash
Butternut squash	Dumpling squash	Cauliflower
Acorn squash	Delicata squash	

2 If you're not using any Veggies for sauce, use 2½ cups total of Cream (if using; it's best with at least ½ cup/70 g cashews in a combination). Transfer to a blender with Aromatics (if using).

Cream ----------- *and/or* ----------→ Aromatics

½ CUP TOTAL
Choose one or combine, or skip altogether

Coconut cream

Raw, unsalted cashews, soaked for 4 to 6 hours, drained, and rinsed

Raw, unsalted, hulled sunflower seeds, soaked for 4 to 6 hours, drained, and rinsed

Raw, unsalted macadamia nuts, unsoaked

Choose one or combine, or skip altogether

¼ cup (40 g) diced onion or shallot, sautéed

1 to 3 garlic cloves, diced and sautéed

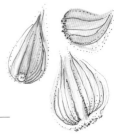

---

3 Add Extras (if using) to the blender, followed by Acid and Funk (if using), the **water, oil** (optional, but adds butteriness), and **salt**. Purée until ultra-smooth, adding more water, ¼ cup (60 ml) at a time, as needed to reach the desired consistency. Season with more salt and **pepper** to taste if you like. Warm the sauce in a pot with roasted or steamed veggies, cooked grains, legumes, beans, noodles, or try it anywhere you'd use a creamy, cheesy sauce (see the following recipes for ideas)!

Extras ----------- *and/or* ----------→ Acid

Choose one or combine, or skip altogether

1 to 6 teaspoons chopped fresh herbs

¼ teaspoon liquid smoke

¼ to ½ cup (40 to 75 g) diced bell pepper (any kind), roasted, sautéed, or grilled

1 to 4 tablespoons seeded, diced chile pepper (any kind), roasted, sautéed, or grilled

¼ to 1 teaspoon chipotle powder

Pinch to ¼ teaspoon cayenne pepper

Fresh-cracked black pepper to taste

¼ to ½ cup (45 to 90 g) seeded, diced tomatoes, roasted, sautéed, or grilled

¼ to 1 teaspoon paprika

¼ to 3 teaspoons Sriracha-style hot sauce

¼ to 3 teaspoons Old Bay Seasoning

1 to 4 tablespoons Supergreen Pesto (page 33)

¼ cup (60 g) salsa

¼ to 3 teaspoons Jamaican jerk seasoning

1 to 4 tablespoons Za'atar spice blend

1 to 4 tablespoons BBQ dry rub

½ to 1 teaspoon whole-grain mustard

¼ to 3 teaspoons chili powder

¼ to 1 teaspoon grated citrus zest

¼ to 3 teaspoons berbere spice

¼ to 3 teaspoons Cajun mix

¼ to 2 teaspoons curry powder

¼ to 2 teaspoons garam masala

1 to 4 tablespoons Chimichurri (page 30)

1 TO 3 TEASPOONS TOTAL
Choose one or combine

Fresh lemon juice

Fresh lime juice

Apple cider vinegar

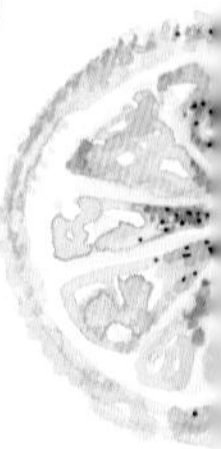

Funk

1 TEASPOON TO 2 TABLESPOONS TOTAL
Choose one or combine, or skip altogether

Nutritional yeast

Pine nuts, toasted

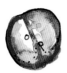

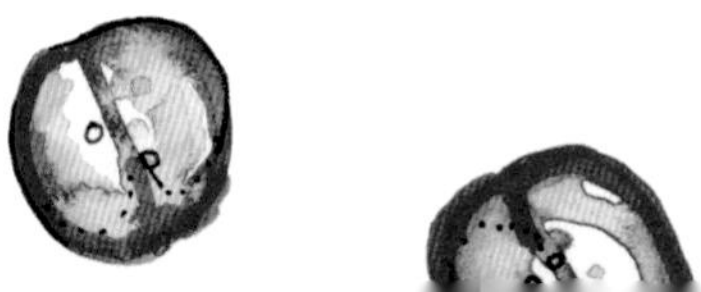

Sriracha Mac

I discovered the magic of Sriracha in my mac and
cheese at a vegan diner in Chicago, and I've been hooked
ever since. For a simple-yet-decadent version,
skip the Sriracha, ginger, and scallions. Try adding
your favorite veggies or switching up the delicata for
sweet potatoes or any other winter squash.

SERVES 4+

One 12-ounce (340 g) package
gluten-free macaroni noodles

2 cups (230 g) peeled,
seeded, and diced delicata
squash, steamed

¾ cup (180 ml) water

½ cup (70 g) raw, unsalted
cashews, soaked for 4 to 6 hours,
drained, and rinsed

1 garlic clove

2 teaspoons fresh lemon juice

2 teaspoons unrefined
coconut oil

1 teaspoon nutritional yeast

1 teaspoon sea salt, plus
more to taste

1 teaspoon Sriracha
(or any similar style hot sauce),
plus more to taste

½ teaspoon peeled, minced fresh
ginger, or ¼ teaspoon ground
ginger (optional)

4 scallions, sliced

Toasted sesame oil (optional)

1   Get a large pot of water boiling and prepare the macaroni noodles according
to the package instructions.

2   While the noodles cook, combine the squash, water, cashews, garlic, lemon
juice, coconut oil, nutritional yeast, salt, Sriracha, and ginger in the blender
and purée until ultra-smooth. Taste and add more Sriracha if you like.
Transfer to a large pot heated to low.

3   Drain the noodles and dump into the pot of sauce; add the scallions.
Stir together, seasoning with more salt if necessary. Drizzle with toasted
sesame oil if you like and serve warm.

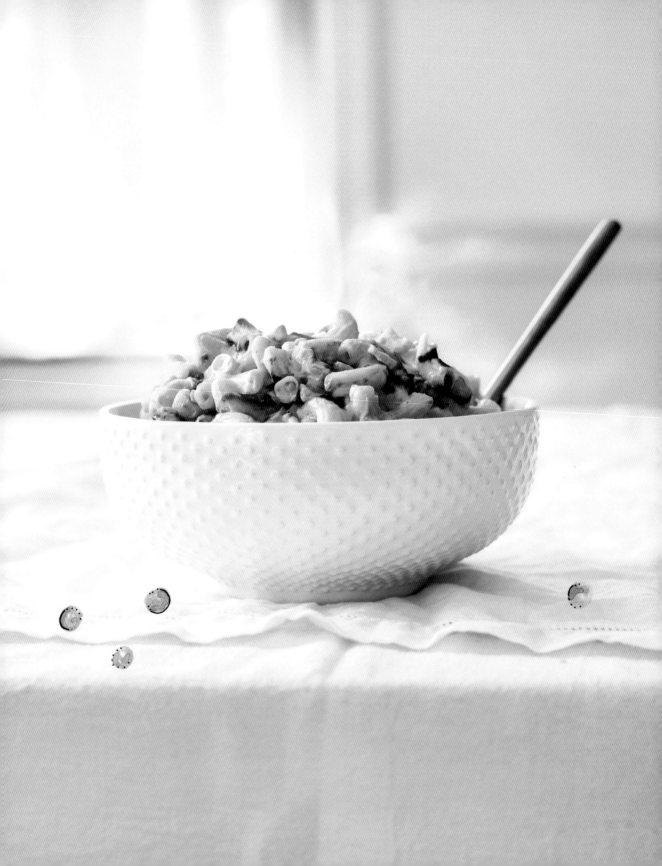

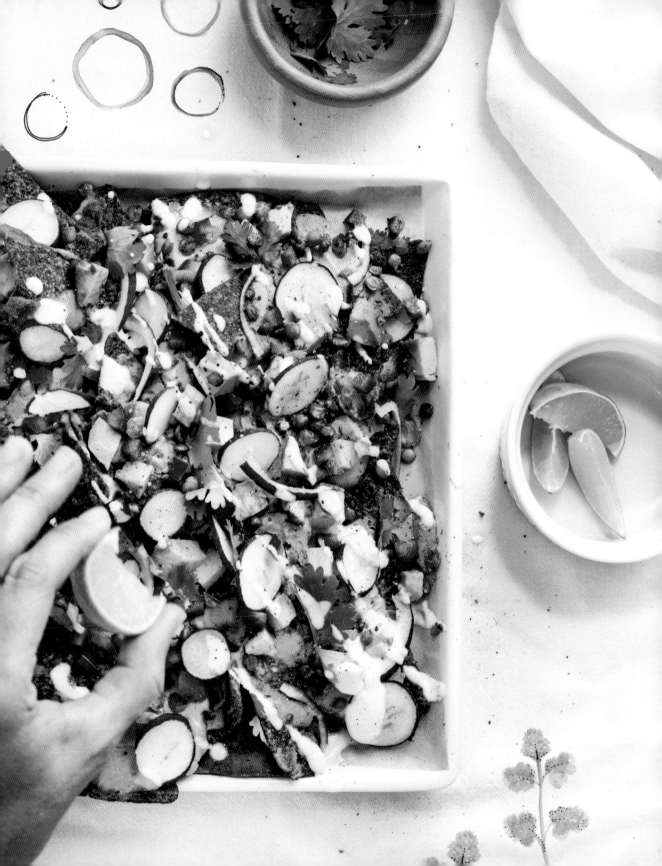

Loaded Nachos

This recipe includes all the fixings so you can have nachos for dinner and feel pretty great about it. Lentils give some protein power to this dish, but you can definitely use black beans, chickpeas, and/or quinoa instead. You can also skip the baking step if you gotta have them right now! This sauce is great on root veggies, noodles, and tacos, too.

SERVES 4+

Veggie Nacho Sauce

1 cup (140 g) peeled, seeded, diced butternut squash, steamed or roasted

½ cup (120 ml) water, plus more if needed

¼ cup (35 g) raw, unsalted cashews, soaked for 4 to 6 hours, drained, and rinsed

1 garlic clove

2 teaspoons nutritional yeast

1 teaspoon apple cider vinegar

1 teaspoon fresh lime juice

1 teaspoon unrefined coconut oil

¾ teaspoon paprika (smoked or plain—chef's choice)

¾ teaspoon sea salt, plus more to taste

¼ teaspoon chipotle powder

—

2 teaspoons unrefined coconut oil

1 cup (200 g) cooked brown lentils (see page 11)

2 teaspoons taco seasoning mix

Sea salt

Fresh-cracked black pepper

5 to 6 large handfuls non-GMO tortilla chips (look for thick and sturdy)

1 avocado, diced

Handful diced red bell pepper

Handful sliced radish

Handful sliced red onion

Handful fresh cilantro leaves

Coconut cream (from a can of coconut milk) or Cashew Cream (page 32) for drizzling (optional)

1. Preheat the oven to 350°F (180°C). Line a baking sheet with unbleached parchment paper.

2. Make the Veggie Nacho Sauce: Combine the squash, water, cashews, garlic, nutritional yeast, vinegar, lime juice, oil, paprika, salt, and chipotle powder in a blender and purée until ultra-smooth. Add more water, 1 tablespoon at a time, until you reach a thick and creamy consistency—not watery. Set aside.

3. In a skillet heated to medium, add the oil and sauté the lentils and taco seasoning for 5 minutes, letting the lentils sear a bit. Season to taste with salt and black pepper.

4. Scatter the chips over the parchment-lined baking sheet and sprinkle with the lentils. Drizzle the nacho sauce on top. Bake for 10 minutes. Remove from the oven and top with the avocado, red pepper, radish, red onion, cilantro, and coconut cream or Cashew Cream (if using), and enjoy.

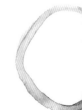

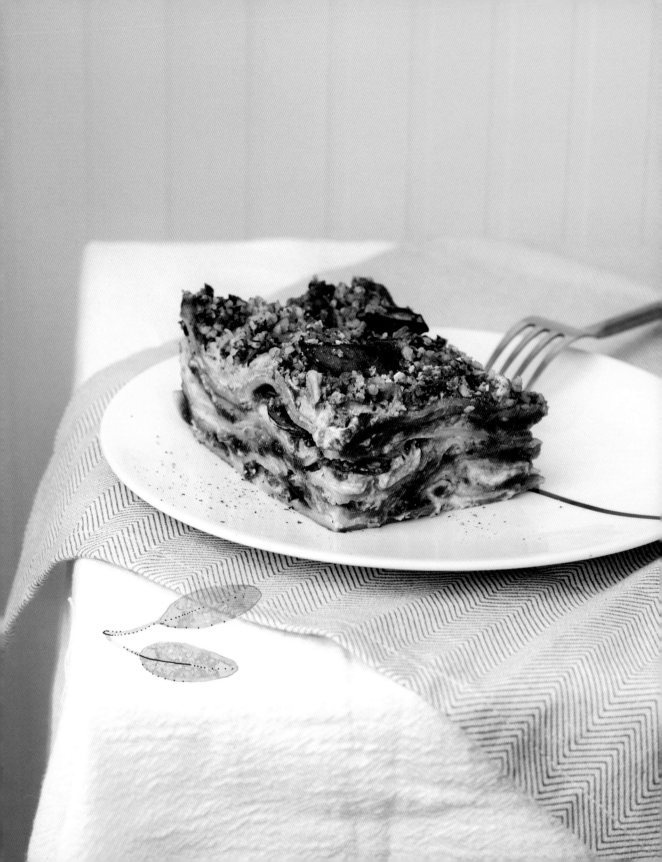

Mushroom & Sage Lasagna

Folks of all dietary inclinations love this comforting recipe.

8+ SERVINGS

½ cup (70 g) raw, unsalted almonds

¼ cup (25 g) raw, unsalted pecans

5 teaspoons unrefined coconut oil

1¼ teaspoons sea salt, plus more to taste

Fresh-cracked black pepper

Pinch fresh-ground nutmeg

3 large leaves kale, chopped into small pieces

One 9-ounce (255 g) package gluten-free lasagna noodles

2½ cups (340 g) cashews, soaked for 4 to 6 hours, drained, and rinsed

1½ cups (360 ml) water

½ cup (65 g) pine nuts, toasted

3 teaspoons fresh lemon juice

5 to 6 sage leaves

1½ pounds (680 g) cremini mushrooms, sliced

2 large shallots, sliced or diced (about 1 cup/80 g)

1 tablespoon Sucanat or coconut palm sugar

2 to 3 tablespoons dry white wine (optional)

1 batch Maudie's Tomato Sauce (page 32), or two 24-ounce (680 g) jars pasta sauce

1. Preheat the oven to 375°F (190°C). In a food processor, pulse together the almonds, pecans, 1 teaspoon of the oil, ¼ teaspoon of the salt, a few grinds of pepper, and the nutmeg until dusty. Add the kale and pulse 3 times.

2. Prepare the noodles according to the package instructions—layer them in rows on sheets of parchment to keep them from sticking to each other.

3. Make a cashew cream sauce by blending the cashews, water, pine nuts, lemon juice, 2 teaspoons of the oil, 1 teaspoon of the salt, and the sage until smooth; set aside.

4. In a skillet heated to medium, add the remaining 2 teaspoons oil, the mushrooms, shallots, Sucanat, and a pinch of salt. Stir occasionally for 7 to 10 minutes, until they caramelize and brown. Add the wine (if using), stir for 2 more minutes or until it cooks off, and remove from the heat.

5. Spread 3 spoonfuls of tomato sauce in a lasagna pan; top with noodles side by side. Spread a few spoonfuls of tomato sauce and cashew cream sauce over the noodles. Sprinkle with the mushrooms, season the layer with a pinch of salt and fresh pepper, then top with another layer of noodles. Repeat these steps, seasoning each layer with a pinch of salt and pepper, until all the noodles, sauces, and mushrooms are used. Sprinkle with the almond-pecan-kale topping, cover with parchment, and bake for 20 minutes. Remove the parchment and bake for 20 more minutes, until bubbling.

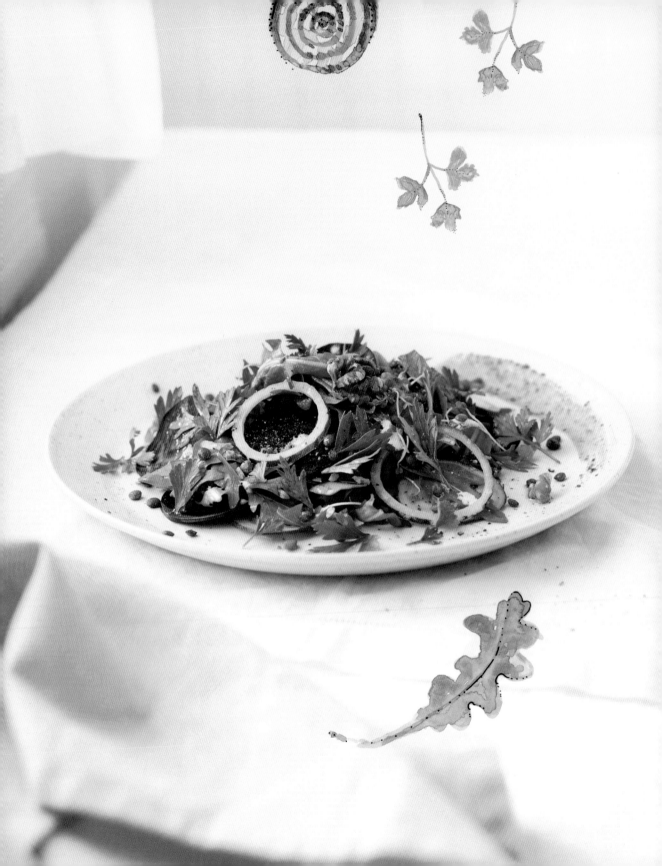

Epic Salads

This template will help you take salads
from "side and starter" status to a craveable,
satisfying main course.

Anyone can make a salad, sure, but do
you know how to make one that's downright
restaurant worthy?

The keys are representing a variety of flavors in
each bowl like salt, sweet, acid, and bitter,
as well as contrasting textures like tender lettuces
with crunchy nuts and chewy dried fruit.

Another secret is sea salt—a simple pinch
enhances flavor and, along with the guidelines
above, helps create a salad so scrumptious
that you want to serve it up in a big mixing bowl
night after night.

Epic Salad combo on this spread:
Beets, toasted walnuts, lentils, parsley, red onion &
Chimichurri (page 30).

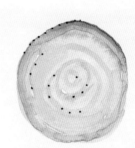

Epic Salads

**2+ SERVINGS
PREP TIME: 15 TO 35 MINUTES**

Use a veggie peeler to shave asparagus, carrots, and summer squash into "noodles." Run hearty main ingredients like cabbage and brussels sprouts over a grater. Throw firm pears, radicchio, and romaine on the grill for some char. Roast veggies like cabbage, beets, onions, eggplant, and winter squash to add comforting flavor and texture to a salad. Use bitter greens like mustard and dandelion sparingly in a mix and, when washing all greens, make sure they are good and dry before using—no soggy lettuce. You can even skip lettuce altogether and try a salad with other main ingredients instead.

Toss delicate leaves gently, and massage the hearty ones like kale. Also, be sure to reference page 26 for more examples of each ingredient group—only a few of many, many options are listed here.

What you need no matter what:

Pinch sea salt, plus more to taste
Fresh-cracked black pepper

Lettuces: Tender, slightly sweet leaves like Bibb, red leaf, spring mix, and Boston love a light and simple Vinaigrette (page 31) or just lemon juice, a splash of oil, and S&P to taste.

Chicories: Bitter, strong leaves that love to dance with creamy, sweet dressings and a pinch of sea salt.

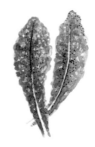

Hearty Greens: Dense leaves that benefit from a quick massage with a little oil and sea salt—this cuts bitterness and softens texture. Chop into small pieces and try with creamy, acidic dressings.

Stronger lettuces like iceberg and romaine can handle fattier, creamy dressings and are also tasty with a simple vinaigrette (since the leaves are so delicate in flavor).

Watercress: Peppery like arugula, but a bit tougher; try watercress with a Vinaigrette (page 31) or a mildly creamy dressing.

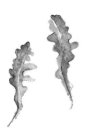

Arugula: Delicate, peppery leaves delicious with a little sweetness (maple, honey) from a light and simple Vinaigrette (page 31) or fruit.

1 In a large bowl, spoon some Dressing (if using) into the bottom of your bowl and fill with Mains. Add a pinch of **salt** and toss gently until thoroughly coated.

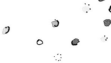

Dressing

1 TO 4 TABLESPOONS TOTAL
Choose one or combine, or skip altogether

Chipotle Cream
(page 28)

Savory Marinade
(page 28)

Orange-Sesame
Sauce (page 30)

Chimichurri
(page 30)

Smoky BBQ Sauce
(page 30)

Supergreen Pesto
(page 33)

Vinaigrette (page 31)

Ranch dressing

Italian dressing

Fresh citrus juice

Balsamic reduction

Goddess dressing

Honey mustard
dressing

Coconut Yogurt
(page 94)

Mains

3 TO 5 CUPS CHOPPED TOTAL
Choose at least two, or more

Lettuces (spring mix,
baby greens, Bibb,
red leaf, romaine)

Tender greens
(arugula, spinach,
watercress)

Hearty greens (kale,
chard, beet greens)

Chicories (endive,
frisée, radicchio)

Brassicas (broccoli,
brussels sprouts,
cabbage, cauliflower)

Roots & tubers
(carrots, beets,
jicama)

Green beans

Mushrooms
(portobello,
button, cremini)

Nightshades
(peppers, tomatoes,
eggplant, potatoes)

Stalks (celery,
asparagus)

Summer squash
(zucchini, yellow
squash, cousa)

Winter squash,
peeled, seeded, and
cooked (butternut,
delicata)

Red onion

Fresh peas
(no need to chop)

Sweet corn kernels
(no need to chop)

---

2 Gently fold in Crunch, Protein, and Special Additions (if using). Season with more salt if needed and **black pepper** to taste.

Crunch ---- *and* ---> Protein

¼ TO ½ CUP TOTAL
Choose one or combine, or skip altogether

Crunchies
(page 145)

Nuts & seeds,
toasted or raw

Croutons

Granola (page 45)

¼ TO 1 CUP
Choose one or
combine, or skip
altogether; page 11
for cooking tips

Chickpeas, cooked

Beans (any kind),
cooked

Buckwheat, cooked

Lentils, cooked

Millet, cooked

Quinoa, cooked

Special Additions

1 TABLESPOON TO ½ CUP TOTAL
Choose one or combine, or skip altogether

Edible flowers
(nasturtiums)

Marinated veggies
(olives, artichokes)

Pickled or fermented
veggies (kimchi,
onions, capers)

Nutritional yeast

Dry or fresh fruit
(pome, berries,
tropical, stone,
cucumber,
avocado, melon)

Toasted coconut

Chopped fresh
herbs (dill, basil,
mint, parsley,
tarragon,
chervil, chives)

Scallions

Cashew-Almond
Cheese Crumbles
(page 133)

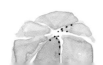
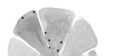

Massaged Kale & Mango Salad *with* Creamy Chipotle Dressing

This is a robust salad that I eat up straight from the mixing bowl because I can't wait to dig in. Nutty quinoa, almonds, and pepitas, plus sweet mango, creamy-cooling avocado, and spicy chipotle dressing are a magical combo. Due to its heartiness, this salad will keep for a day or two (yep, even dressed) in the fridge.

SERVES 2+

¼ cup (35 g) raw, unsalted almonds

¼ cup (30 g) raw, unsalted pepitas

Two pinches plus ¼ teaspoon sea salt, plus more to taste

¼ cup (60 ml) Chipotle Cream (page 28; fridge or freeze any extra)

3 teaspoons extra virgin olive oil

1 to 3 tablespoons water

5 cups (80 g) lightly packed stemmed, chopped kale (any kind)

½ cup (90 g) cooked tricolor or black quinoa (roughly 2 tablespoons dry; see page 11)

½ cup (75 g) diced avocado

½ cup (85 g) diced mango

¼ cup (30 g) thinly sliced red onion

1 lime

Handful fresh cilantro leaves

1   Preheat the oven to 350°F (180°C). Line a baking sheet with unbleached parchment paper and spread the almonds and pepitas in one layer on the sheet so they have room to toast mostly untouched on all sides. Sprinkle with a pinch of salt and pop in the oven for 7 minutes. Remove from the baking sheet, chop roughly, and set aside to cool.

2   In a small bowl, whisk together the Chipotle Cream, 2 teaspoons of the oil, and the water until you get a pourable dressing consistency. Set aside.

3   Place the kale in a large mixing bowl, drizzle with the remaining 1 teaspoon oil, and the ¼ teaspoon salt. Use your hands to massage and squeeze the kale for 2 to 3 minutes, until the leaves darken and become tender.

4   Pour 2 tablespoons of the dressing into the bottom of the bowl and gently toss with the kale, quinoa, avocado, mango, onion, and a small pinch of salt. Top with a generous squeeze of fresh lime juice, the cilantro, and toasted pepitas and almonds. Add more salt and dressing to taste.

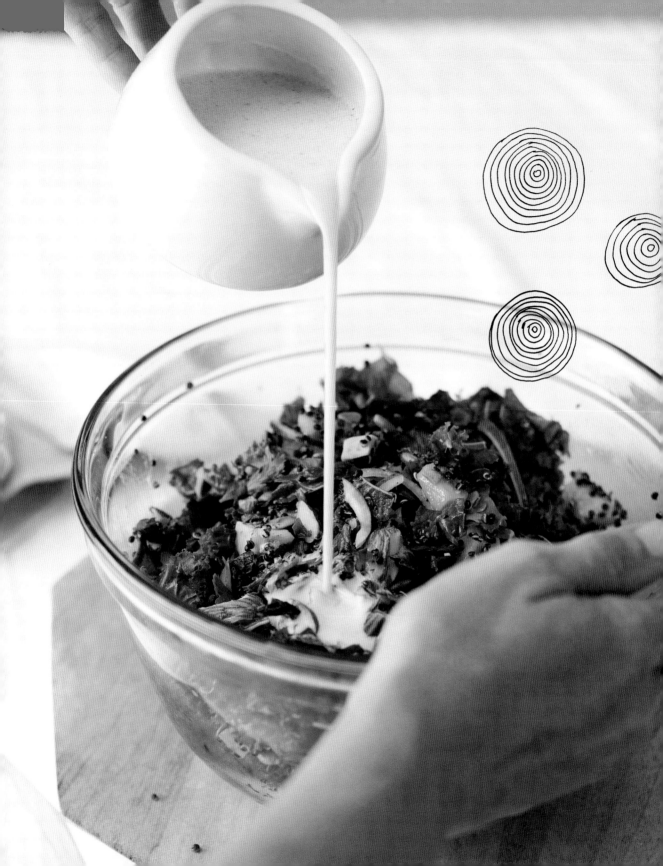

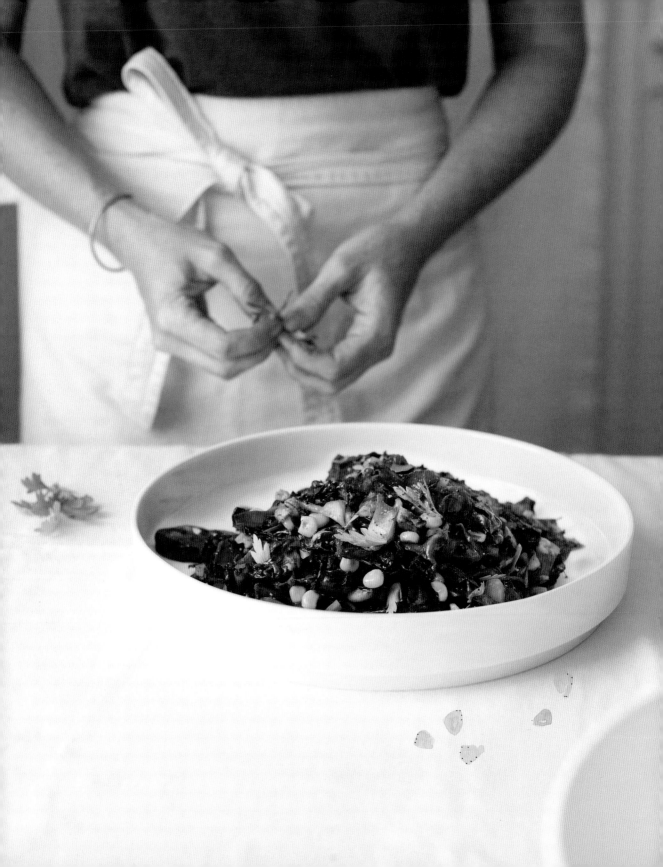

Roasted Cabbage & Sweet Corn Salad *with* Honey Mustard Vinaigrette

Crunchy, oven-roasted cabbage with sweet pops of corn, bright-fresh parsley, and a sweet-sour honey mustard vinaigrette riff from page 31—this is an Epic Salad. Char the cabbage and corn on the grill for extra flavor.

SERVES 2+

Grapeseed oil

1 small head purple or green cabbage (or a combination of both)

Two pinches sea salt, or more to taste

Fresh-cracked black pepper

½ cup (75 g) sweet corn kernels

¼ cup (30 g) thinly sliced or diced red onion

A large handful chopped fresh parsley

—

Honey Mustard Vinaigrette (from page 31 formula)

3 tablespoons extra virgin olive oil

2 tablespoons apple cider vinegar

1 tablespoon minced shallot

2 teaspoons raw, unpasteurized honey

1½ teaspoons whole-grain or Dijon mustard

Pinch sea salt

1. Preheat the oven to 375°F (190°C) and lightly grease a baking dish with the oil. Starting at the top of the head, slice the cabbage into ¼-inch (6 mm) pieces and lay them in the baking dish. Drizzle each with a little bit of oil and season with a pinch of salt and generous pepper. Roast for 40 to 45 minutes, until the center is tender and the edges start to brown and crisp. Remove from the oven, cool for a few minutes until it's comfy to handle, and chop into large bite-sized pieces. Transfer to a large bowl.

2. Toss the corn into a dry skillet heated to medium and allow the kernels to sear for 1 to 2 minutes—give the skillet a shake and sear for 1 to 2 minutes more. Add to the bowl with the cabbage.

3. Meanwhile, make the Honey Mustard Vinaigrette: Whisk the ingredients together in a small bowl.

4. Add a few tablespoons of vinaigrette to the bowl with the cabbage and corn. Toss with the onion, parsley, a small pinch of salt, and black pepper to taste. Add more vinaigrette 1 tablespoon at a time until it tastes perfect to you.

Pesto Panzanella Salad

A bit of a departure from the traditional Italian bread salad,
this particular creation is full of added bright flavor
from peppery arugula and fresh, colorful heirloom tomatoes.
I'll sometimes add a chopped Granny Smith apple for
bites of vibrant tartness.

SERVES 1 TO 2

2 cups (70 g) cubed day-old
gluten-free bread

¼ cup (35 g) raw, unsalted
pine nuts

1 cup (180 g) chopped
heirloom tomatoes

1 cup (25 g) packed arugula

¼ cup (35 g) chopped cucumber

¼ cup (40 g) chopped red
or yellow bell pepper

¼ cup (30 g) thinly sliced
red onion

Pinch sea salt, or more
to taste

Fresh-cracked black pepper

Pesto Vinaigrette

½ cup (120 ml) Supergreen Pesto
(page 33) or store-bought

2 tablespoons red wine vinegar

1 garlic clove, minced

1 teaspoon raw, unpasteurized
honey (optional)

Extra virgin olive oil for
drizzling (optional)

1. Preheat the oven to 300°F (150°C). Lay out the bread cubes on a baking
   sheet and bake for 15 to 20 minutes, until crispy on the outside and soft
   in the middle (alternatively, you can leave them out overnight to harden).
   Transfer to a large bowl.

2. Spread the pine nuts on the baking sheet and toast for 7 to 10 minutes,
   until starting to brown. Add them to the bowl, along with the tomatoes,
   arugula, cucumber, bell pepper, onion, salt, and black pepper to taste.

3. Whisk together all the vinaigrette ingredients until smooth. Pour into
   the bowl and toss well. Drizzle with extra olive oil if you like and serve.

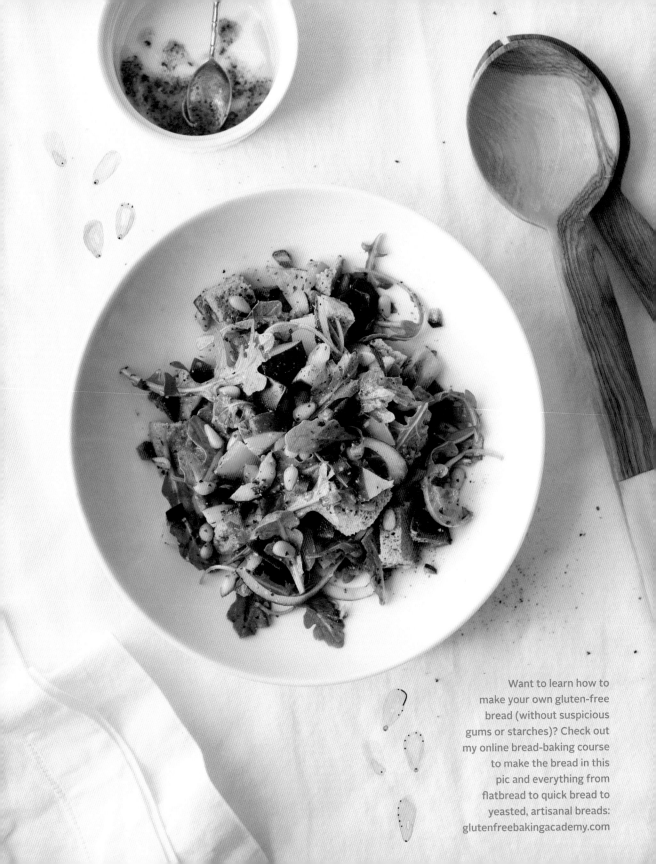

Want to learn how to make your own gluten-free bread (without suspicious gums or starches)? Check out my online bread-baking course to make the bread in this pic and everything from flatbread to quick bread to yeasted, artisanal breads: glutenfreebakingacademy.com

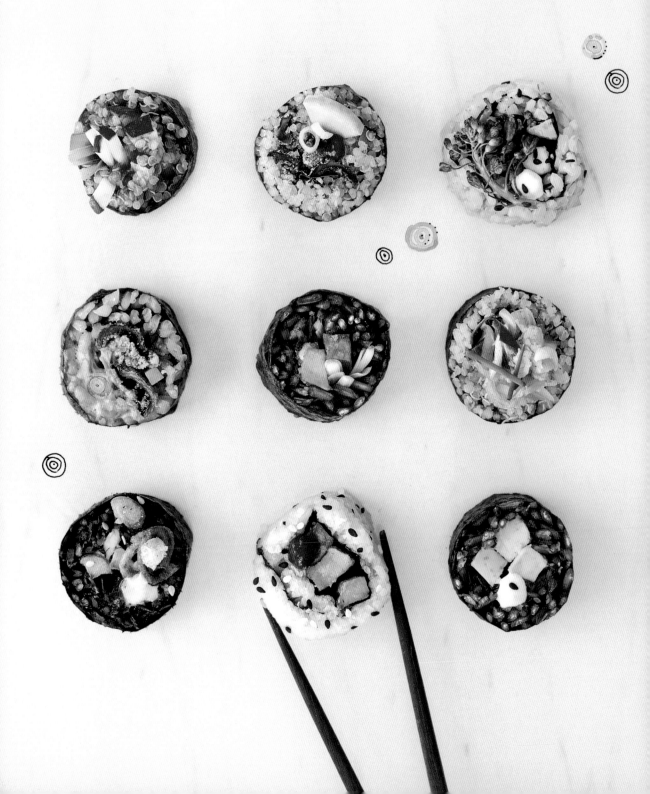

Mmmaki

Veggie sushi makis (cut rolls) are perfect for
pantry-to-plate cooking because you just need a few sheets
of nori, some cooked rice or quinoa, a handful of
veggies, and a smidge of imagination to whip up a
creative meal in minutes.

Try hearty roasted veg for a substantial, umami filling,
or seafood-textured mushrooms (lobster, oyster,
or lion's mane) sautéed in some oil, a little garlic, and
a pinch of sea salt. Go for fresh and simple, or
creamy and rich combos.

You also don't need any fancy mats or tools
to make maki at home—just some plastic wrap
(makes for nonstick rolling) and a dish towel.
If you end up with any extra filling—
hey, Scrambles (page 36) or an Epic Salad
(page 195) for dinner tomorrow!

The recipes I share here demonstrate some
fun techniques, but by all means, a simple avocado
and cucumber roll hits the spot, too.

Mmmaki combos on this spread starting top left to right:
Sriracha-quinoa, radish & scallion; crispy mushroom, carrot & quinoa; roasted broccoli,
avocado, cucumber, brown rice & miso mayo; crispy shiitake, yellow pepper,
scallion & sriracha mayo; sprouted red rice, miso-roasted sweet potato & scallion;
quinoa & Fire Breathin' Fermented Veggies (page 157); Midnight Maki (page 213);
Sticky "Jade Pearl" Rice (page 209), steamed sweet potato & sriracha;
sprouted red rice, avocado & garlic mayo.

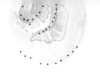

Mmmaki

MAKES 3 TO 4 MAKI
PREP TIME: 15 TO 30 MINUTES

For gluten-free "tempura like" preparation ideas, see page 210—
you can use those tips for pretty much all veggies. And to make a
Sushi Mayo, simply use Cashew Cream from page 32 as a base
and stir in 1 to 3 teaspoons of any of the following to taste: roasted
garlic, chipotle powder or adobo sauce, citrus juice and/or grated
zest (lemon, lime, orange, yuzu, kumquat, blood orange), Sriracha,
wasabi powder, Dijon or whole-grain mustard, Old Bay, herbs
(cilantro, chives, basil, mint), miso, toasted sesame oil, truffle
oil, or sautéed onion.

What you need no matter what:

3 or 4 nori sheets (dried seaweed)

1 batch Sticky Rice (page 209)
or quinoa

Small dish of water

Wasabi (optional)

Coconut aminos, tamari, or soy sauce for dipping (optional)

1 Lay down a bamboo mat or clean dish towel folded to about 8 x 10 inches (20 x 25 cm) in front of you on a countertop so the short side is parallel to your belly. Lay a similarly sized piece of plastic wrap on top of the mat or towel. Place a sheet of **nori** shiny side down on top of the plastic wrap. Starting with the edge closest to you, spoon **Sticky Rice** onto the nori ¼ inch (6 mm) thick, not packing it down but gently covering the sheet. Work away from your belly and fill the sheet only three-quarters full of rice—leave an inch or two (2.5 to 5 cm) of the far end of the nori free from rice.

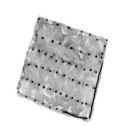

2 On top of the rice, and on the edge closest to you, lay a row of Main Filling (if using) left to right, about 1 inch (2.5 cm) wide. On top of the Main Filling, lay a row of Fresh ½ to 1 inch (1 to 2.5 cm) wide, then lay a row of Creamy (if using) in front of them about ¼ inch (6 mm). Lift the edge of the bamboo mat or towel nearest you and fold it over the fillings—give it a gentle squeeze. With a careful rolling motion and steady pressure, continue rolling, creating a cylinder. When you've almost rolled to the end, dip your finger in the **dish of water** and run it along the un-riced edge of nori, then complete your roll and gently squeeze into a cylinder, using the plastic wrap to help you shape it.

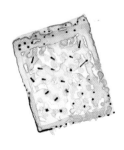

Main Filling ---- *and/or* ---> Fresh

2 CUPS CHOPPED TOTAL

Choose one or combine or skip altogether;
raw, roasted, or steamed

Broccoli

Cauliflower

Carrots

Beets

Green beans

Mushrooms

Eggplant

Asparagus

Summer squash

Winter squash,
peeled, seeded,
and cooked

Potatoes

Sweet potatoes

Bell pepper (any)

2 CUPS CHOPPED TOTAL

Choose one

Jicama

Cucumber

Green apple

Carrots

Bell pepper

Red onion

Fresh peas
(no need to chop)

Sweet corn kernels
(no need to chop)

Scallions

Fresh herbs

Creamy

½ CUP TOTAL

Choose one or combine or skip altogether

Cashew Cream
(page 32)

Chipotle Cream
(page 28)

Sushi Mayo
(any of the ideas
from the intro, left)

Probiotic
Cream Cheese
(page 128)

Avocado, sliced

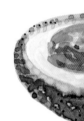

3 Remove the plastic wrap from the nori and place the roll on a cutting board. With a very
sharp chef's knife, slice the maki in the center, then slice the two halves in half, and repeat
until you get even slices—about 6 to 8 depending on the size you want. Follow these steps
again to make 2 to 3 more makis, then garnish with Toppings, and if you like, serve with
wasabi and a small dipping dish filled with **coconut aminos, tamari, or soy sauce.**

Toppings

Choose one or combine, or skip altogether

1 avocado, sliced
or diced

2 to 4 tablespoons
Cashew Cream
(page 32)

2 to 4 tablespoons
Chipotle Cream
(page 28)

2 to 4 tablespoons
Sushi Mayo (any
of the ideas from
the intro, left)

1 tablespoon toasted
sesame seeds

1 to 3 tablespoons
chopped toasted
nuts and/or seeds

1 to 3 teaspoons
Sriracha

1 to 4 tablespoons
fresh herbs

1 to 3 teaspoons
sliced scallions

2 to 4 tablespoons
fried sliced shallot
(page 213)

1 to 2 teaspoons
toasted sesame oil

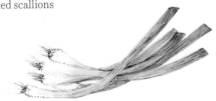

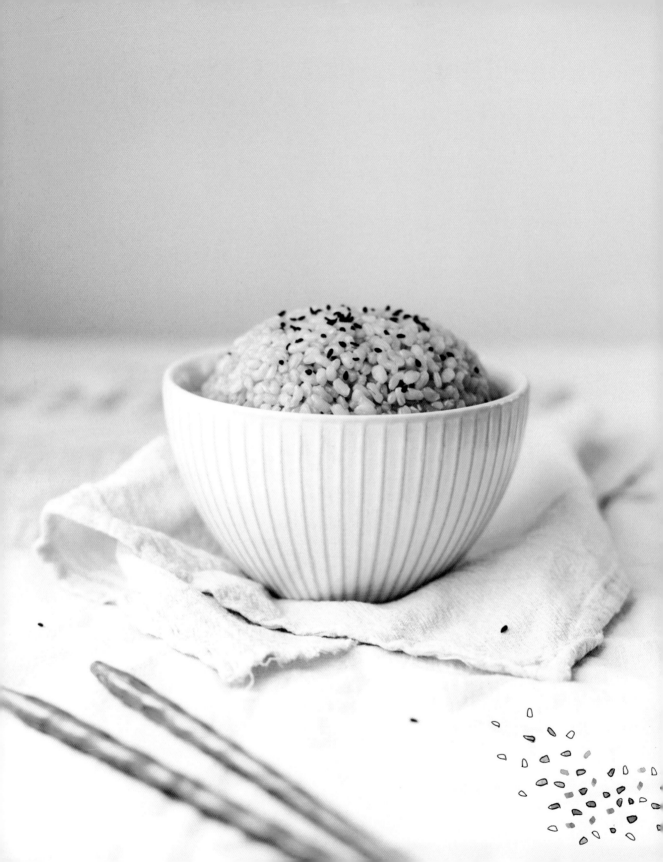

Sticky Rice

This recipe is a template in itself—it walks you through the steps to make sticky brown rice for scrumptious Mmmaki making, but you can sub the amounts of rice called for here in equal amounts with gold quinoa for Sticky Quinoa—just check out page 11 for cooking tips and water amounts. You can also try any other variety of rice like sprouted rice, black rice, red rice, basmati, or bamboo rice—just skip the processed white stuff; you get more flavor and nutrients with others.

MAKES 2½ TO 3 CUPS (510 TO 615 G) STICKY RICE, ENOUGH FOR 3 OR 4 MAKI

---

1 cup (180 g) short-grain brown rice

3 cups (720 ml) water for cooking, plus more for rinsing

2 tablespoons rice wine vinegar

2 tablespoons Sucanat or coconut sugar

Pinch sea salt

---

1. Place the rice in a large bowl and fill it with water so the rice is covered. Swish the rice with your hands back and forth 20 to 30 times (there's something so relaxing about this). Drain, rinse, and repeat (ahhh). Drain and rinse again until the water runs clear, then transfer the rice to a pot. Fill with the 3 cups (720 ml) water and bring to a boil. Once boiling, reduce the heat to a simmer and cover with a lid to cook for 20 to 30 minutes—until the water is absorbed and the grains are soft yet firm, not mushy when tasted. Remove from the heat, keep the lid on, and let sit for 10 minutes—try not to peek; that steam helps make fluffy, sticky heaven.

2. Meanwhile, whisk together the vinegar, Sucanat, and salt until dissolved.

3. Spoon the rice into a large mixing bowl and pour the vinegar mixture on top. Cut through the rice with a wooden spoon until evenly distributed and allow the rice to cool to room temperature.

Dynamite Mushroom Maki

You can swap out many veggies for mushrooms here—
the crispy brown rice cereal gives it all a panko-like crumb. Use
leftover Sriracha Mayo for an Epic Salad (page 195) dressing.

MAKES 3 TO 4 MAKI

1 cup (30 g) crispy brown rice cereal

2 tablespoons blanched almond flour

2 tablespoons gluten-free all-purpose flour

¼ teaspoon sea salt

2 cups (190 g) mushrooms (white button, baby bella, beech, shiitake)

2 tablespoons unrefined coconut oil, gently warmed to liquid

1 avocado, sliced

4 to 6 scallions, cut into 3-inch (7.5 cm) lengths

3 or 4 nori sheets

1 batch short-grain brown Sticky Rice (page 209)

1 tablespoon toasted sesame seeds

Simple Sriracha Mayo

½ cup (70 g) raw, unsalted cashews, soaked for 4 to 6 hours, drained, and rinsed

¼ cup (60 ml) water

1 teaspoon Sriracha (or similar style hot sauce), plus more to taste

Two pinches sea salt or more to taste

1 Preheat the oven to 400°F (200°C) and line a baking sheet with unbleached parchment paper.

2 Blend together all the Sriracha Mayo ingredients and taste. If you want more heat, blend in 1 to 2 more teaspoons of Sriracha and set aside.

3 In a food processor, pulse the crispy brown rice cereal, flours, and salt until broken up but still maintaining a bit of texture. You can also put the cereal in a bag and use your hands to pulverize. Set aside.

4 Wipe the mushrooms clean with a dry towel and slice into large pieces—transfer to a bowl with the oil. Toss until the mushrooms are covered, then add the flour-cereal mixture and toss until the mushrooms are coated. Scatter in one layer on a baking sheet—pressing any extra flour mixture onto the mushrooms—and bake for 25 minutes. Remove from the oven, flip, and bake for another 10 minutes, or until crispy and brown. Set aside.

5 Divide the avocado, scallions, and mushrooms into three or four portions, depending on how many maki you want to make. Then follow steps 1 to 3 on template page 206 to roll each maki with a portion of mushrooms, avocado, scallions, and Sriracha Mayo inside. Slice and serve topped with Sriracha Mayo and toasted sesame seeds.

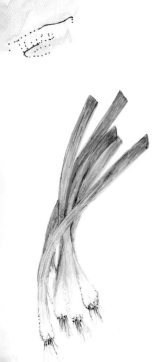

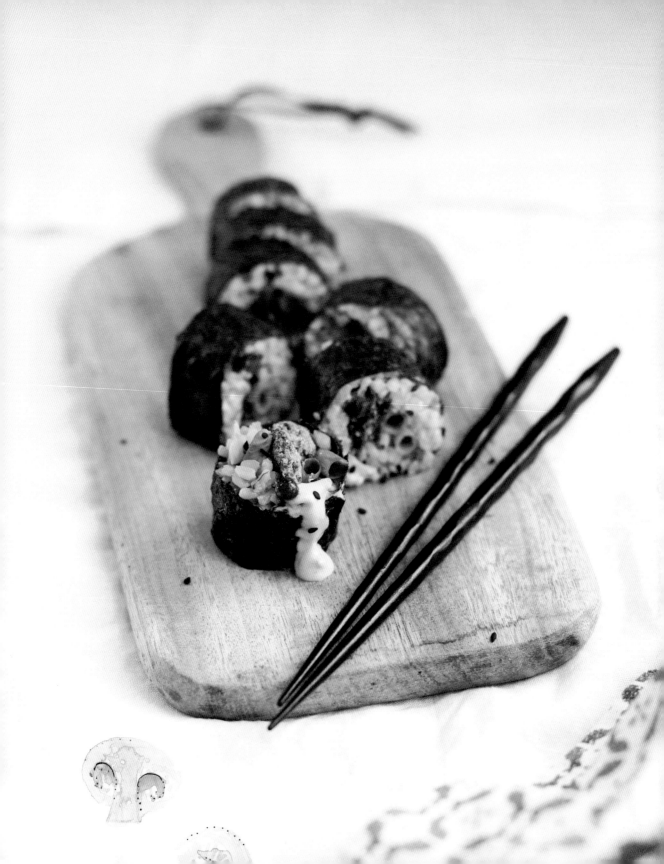

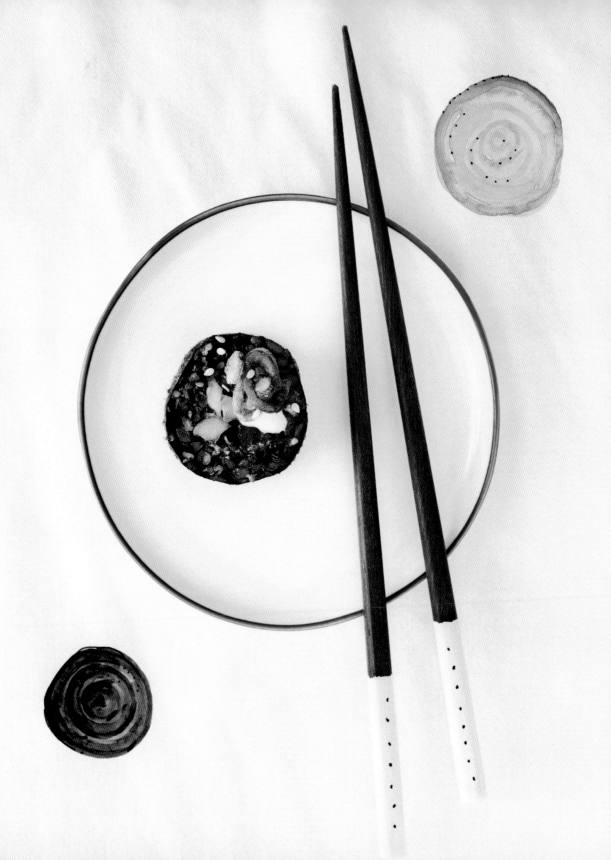

Midnight Maki

This maki benefits from marinating, so plan ahead, but you can roast the veggies in the marinade right away. Use leftover Savory Marinade or Roasted Garlic Mayo for an Epic Salad (page 195) dressing.

MAKES 3 TO 4 MAKI

1 cup (135 g) peeled, sliced red beets (cut into 2-inch/5 cm matchsticks)

1 cup (130 g) peeled, sliced yellow or orange carrots (cut into 2-inch/5 cm matchsticks)

1 batch Savory Marinade (page 28)

1 tablespoon gluten-free all-purpose flour

A few pinches sea salt

Fresh-cracked black pepper

1 shallot, thinly sliced

½ cup (120 ml) grapeseed or avocado oil

1 avocado, sliced

2 to 4 radishes, sliced into matchsticks

3 or 4 nori sheets

1 batch black Sticky Rice (page 209)

Toasted sesame seeds

Roasted Garlic Mayo

½ cup (70 g) raw, unsalted cashews, soaked for 4 to 6 hours, drained, and rinsed

¼ cup (60 ml) water

1 teaspoon fresh lemon juice

2 garlic cloves, roasted

Two pinches sea salt, or more to taste

1. In a roasting dish, scatter the beets and carrots in one layer and pour the Savory Marinade on top. Stir a bit, cover, and pop in the fridge to marinate for 12 to 24 hours.

2. When you're ready to make the maki, blend together all the Roasted Garlic Mayo ingredients and set aside.

3. In a small bowl, stir together the flour, a pinch of salt, and a few grinds of black pepper. Stir in the shallot and toss until thoroughly coated with flour, then lay out a small plate lined with a paper towel and preheat the oven to 350°F (180°C).

4. In a small pot, heat the oil over medium heat. Use a fork or slotted spoon to gently lower the shallots into the oil. Stir occasionally for 7 to 10 minutes, until they are just starting to brown. Quickly lift them out and transfer to the towel-lined plate. Sprinkle with a pinch of salt.

5. Roast the marinated roots for 20 to 30 minutes, until easily pierced with a fork but firm, not mushy. Divide the roots, avocado, and radishes into three or four portions, depending on how many maki you want. Then follow steps 1 to 3 on template page 206 to roll each maki with a portion of roots, avocado, radishes, and Garlic Mayo inside. Slice and serve topped with more Garlic Mayo, fried shallots, and toasted sesame seeds.

Green Spirit Maki

This fresh and spicy maki is great with brown Sticky Rice or Sticky Quinoa (page 209), so give both a try. If you can't get your hands on any jicama, use Granny Smith apple, zucchini, or even a roasted potato instead.

MAKES 3 TO 4 MAKI

1 avocado, sliced

½ cup (60 g) sliced cucumber (cut into larger matchsticks)

½ cup (60 g) sliced jicama (cut into matchsticks)

1 large jalapeño pepper, seeds and ribs removed, sliced into matchsticks

¼ cup (5 g) packed fresh cilantro, plus more for garnish

3 or 4 nori sheets

1 batch short-grain brown Sticky Rice (page 209)

Juice of 1 lime

Wasabi Mayo

½ cup (70 g) cashews, soaked for 4 to 6 hours, drained, and rinsed

¼ cup (60 ml) water

1½ teaspoons wasabi powder, or more to taste

1 teaspoon coconut aminos (soy sauce or tamari)

1 teaspoon fresh lime juice (reserved from the lime used to garnish the maki)

¼ teaspoon toasted sesame oil

Two pinches sea salt or more to taste

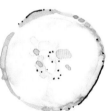

1   Combine all the Wasabi Mayo ingredients in a blender, purée until velvety, and taste. Blend in more wasabi powder ½ teaspoon at a time if you want more kick, then set aside.

2   Divide the avocado, cucumber, jicama, jalapeño, and cilantro into three or four portions, depending on how many maki you want to make. Then follow steps 1 to 3 on template page 206 to roll each maki with a portion of the veggies, cilantro, and Wasabi Mayo inside. Slice and serve topped with some lime juice, more Wasabi Mayo, and a cilantro leaf.

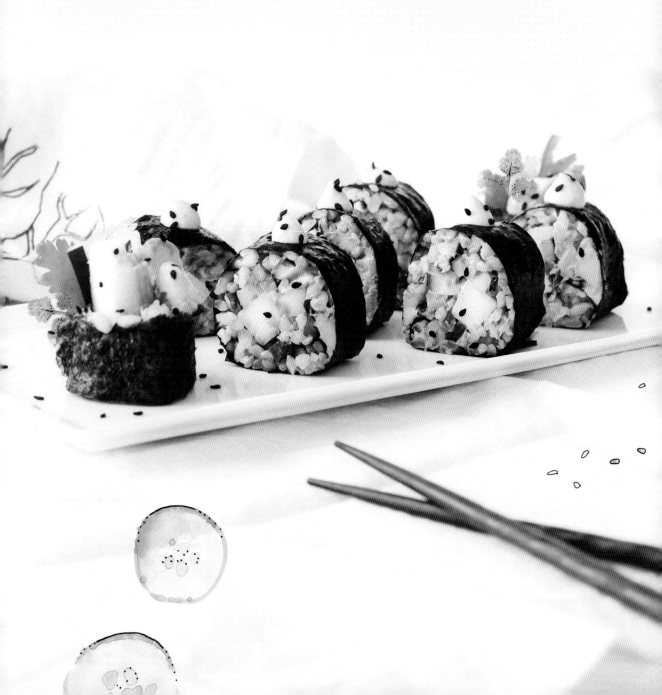

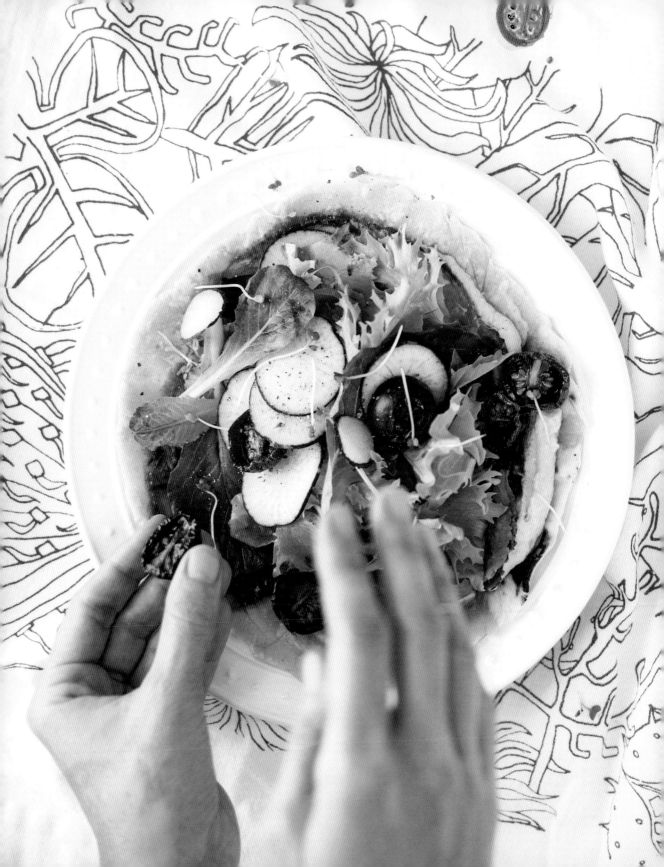

Learn how to make a variety of homemade,
gluten-free tortillas and wraps like the one shown here:
glutenfreebakingacademy.com

Tacos & Wraps

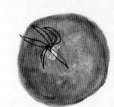

It all starts with a good tortilla or wrap. And if
you have veg in the house, some cooked
grains or beans, and a little sauce, Dip (page 137),
or salsa of some kind, you can make a tasty
meal in minutes.

Use what you have on hand—be sure to marry a
variety of textures like comforting, fresh,
rich, and chewy. Use a good balance of spice,
cooling ingredients, crunch, and freshness.

Try collard greens or Boston lettuce for raw wraps.
Source non-GMO corn ingredients if possible.
And note that mushrooms and small grains will
yield less filling than dense veggies and
beans, so don't be afraid to double batches.

When filling, resist the urge to overload, and
don't forget the toppings!

Wrap combo on this spread:
Roasted tomato, spring greens, hummus, harissa, broccoli
sprouts, radish & cassava flour tortilla.

Tacos & Wraps

2 TO 6 SERVINGS
COOK TIME:
15 TO 35 MINUTES

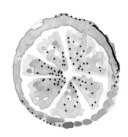

What you need no matter what:

2 teaspoons coconut or grapeseed oil

¼ teaspoon sea salt, or more to taste

1 to 3 garlic cloves, minced (optional)

1   In a skillet heated to medium-high, add the **oil** and sauté Base and Veggies (if using) for 5 to 10 minutes.

Base ---------- *and/or* ----------→ Veggies

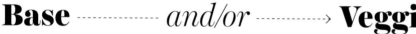

3 CUPS TOTAL

Choose one or combine; page 11 cooking tips for grains and legumes

Winter squash, seeded, diced, and cooked

Summer squash, diced

Cauliflower florets or "rice"

Broccoli florets

Chickpeas, cooked

Lentils, cooked

Buckwheat, cooked

Quinoa, cooked

Mushrooms, chopped

Black beans, cooked

Millet, cooked

Sweet potatoes, diced and cooked

Choose one or combine, or skip altogether

1 cup packed hearty greens

½ to 1 poblano pepper, seeded and diced

1 red bell pepper, seeded and diced or sliced

½ to 1 jalapeño pepper, seeded and diced

1 small onion (any) or shallot, diced

---

2   Sprinkle Spice into your Base and Veggies with the **salt** to taste.
Add the **garlic** if you like; sauté for 3 minutes. Cover and set aside.

Spice Choose one, fresh or store-bought

2 tablespoons BBQ dry rub

2 tablespoons Cajun seasoning

1 tablespoon garam masala

¼ to ½ teaspoon liquid smoke

½ to 1 teaspoon smoked paprika

2 tablespoons za'atar spice blend

1 to 2 tablespoons Jamaican jerk seasoning

1 to 2 tablespoons Montreal steak seasoning

1 to 2 tablespoons Old Bay Seasoning

2 tablespoons taco/ fajita seasoning

3 Warm Tortillas & Wraps in a steamer, on a low gas flame, or in a dry skillet until softened. Layer on a plate (Tip: A piece of parchment between each keeps them from sticking) and cover with a towel to keep warm. For crispy shells, prepare tacos according to the package instructions. For collards, score or remove the stem so you can roll it up (quickly blanch/steam and dry leaves to soften and remove bitterness), or use lettuce leaves for taco shells. Add a few spoonfuls of Base and Veggies to the Tortillas/Wraps.

Tortillas & Wraps

4 TO 8 TOTAL
Choose one

Brown rice tortillas

Corn tortillas

Crispy taco shells

Collard greens

Large Boston lettuce leaves

---

4 Add a drizzle or sprinkle of Cool & Creamy (if using) and a spoonful of Sauce (if using), then top with a little Sour & Acid (if using), and finish with some Fresh (if using).

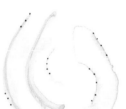

Cool & Creamy

½ TO 1 CUP TOTAL
Choose one or combine, or skip altogether

Mango, diced or sliced

Avocado, diced, mashed, or sliced

Hummus

Coconut Yogurt (page 94)

Cashew Cream (page 32)

Probiotic Cream Cheese (page 129)

Sauce

¼ TO ½ CUP (60 TO 120 ML) TOTAL
Choose one or combine, or skip altogether

Smoky BBQ Sauce (page 30)

Chipotle Cream (page 28)

Hot sauce

Harissa (jar)

Cauliflower Cream (page 32)

Savory Marinade (page 28)

Enchilada Sauce (page 31)

Supergreen Pesto (page 33)

Chimichurri (page 30)

Sour & Acid

Choose one or combine, or skip altogether

Pickled vegetables (onion, peppers, carrots; page 223)

Fermented Veggies (page 153)

Fresh citrus juice

Salsa

Fresh

Choose one or combine, or skip altogether

Fresh herbs

Lettuces (spring mix, arugula)

Sprouts

Fresh corn kernels

Cucumber, sliced or diced

Red onion, diced

Apple, diced

Cucumber, diced

Cabbage, shredded

Peppers (jalapeño, bell, poblano), seeded and diced

Carrots, shredded

Summer squash, diced

Radish, sliced thinly into rounds or matchsticks

Scallions, sliced

Tomatoes, diced

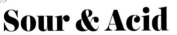

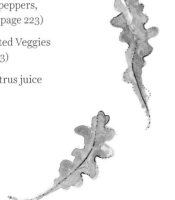
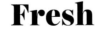
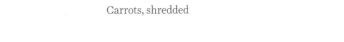

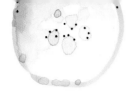

Za'atar-Spiced Lentil Wrap

Za'atar is a Middle Eastern spice blend that's floral and herby—delicious with roasted veggies, cooked legumes, and Crackers (page 112), or even stirred into fresh, unsweetened Coconut Yogurt (page 94).

SERVES 2 TO 3

2 teaspoons unrefined coconut oil, grapeseed oil, or avocado oil

3 cups (600 g) cooked green or brown lentils (roughly 1 cup/190 g dry; see page 11)

1 red bell pepper, ribs removed, seeded, and diced

1 shallot, minced

1 garlic clove, minced

2 tablespoons za'atar spice blend

¼ teaspoon sea salt, plus more to taste

Handful fresh parsley

1 small lemon

5 to 6 gluten-free tortillas/wraps

1 cup (245 g) hummus

½ cup (15 g) arugula

½ cup (65 g) diced cucumber

½ cup (90 g) diced tomatoes

1. In a skillet heated medium, add the oil and sauté the lentils, pepper, and shallot for 5 to 7 minutes, until they start to brown. Add the garlic, za'atar, salt, and half of the parsley (save half for garnish)—cook and stir for 2 to 3 more minutes. Try a spoonful, season with more salt if needed, and squeeze some fresh lemon juice into the mix to taste. Cover with a lid and set aside.

2. Warm the tortillas in a steamer, on a low gas flame, or in a dry skillet until softened. Layer them on a plate (Tip: A small piece of unbleached parchment layered between keeps them from sticking) and cover with a towel to keep warm as you work.

3. Spread a large spoonful of hummus on the bottom of a wrap. Add a few spoonfuls of the lentil mix, followed by 2 to 3 tablespoons each of arugula, cucumber, parsley, and tomatoes. Fold up the two opposite ends of your wrap and hold them down while you lift one of the unfolded sides and roll across to close your wrap. Repeat with other tortillas until all are used. Enjoy warm.

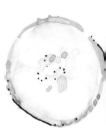

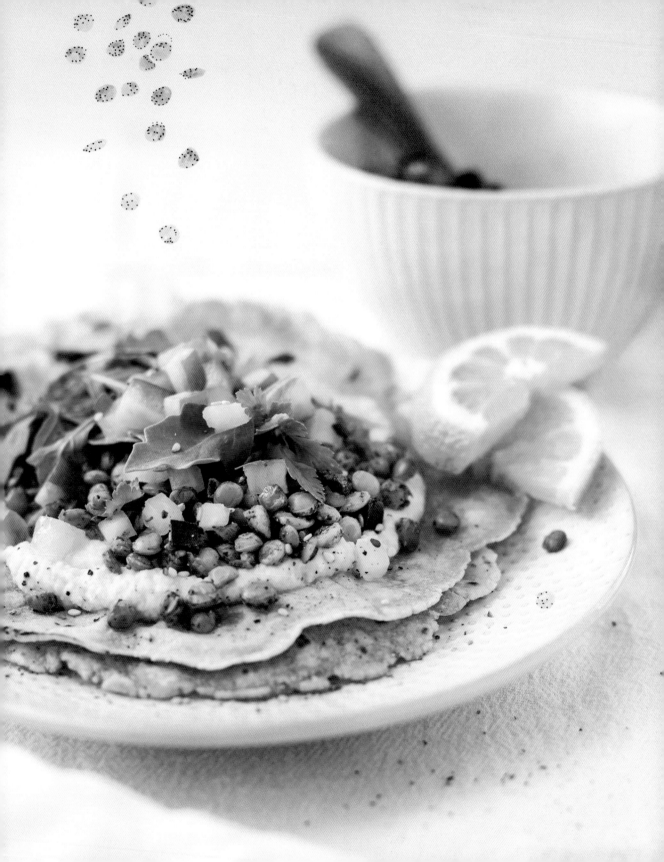

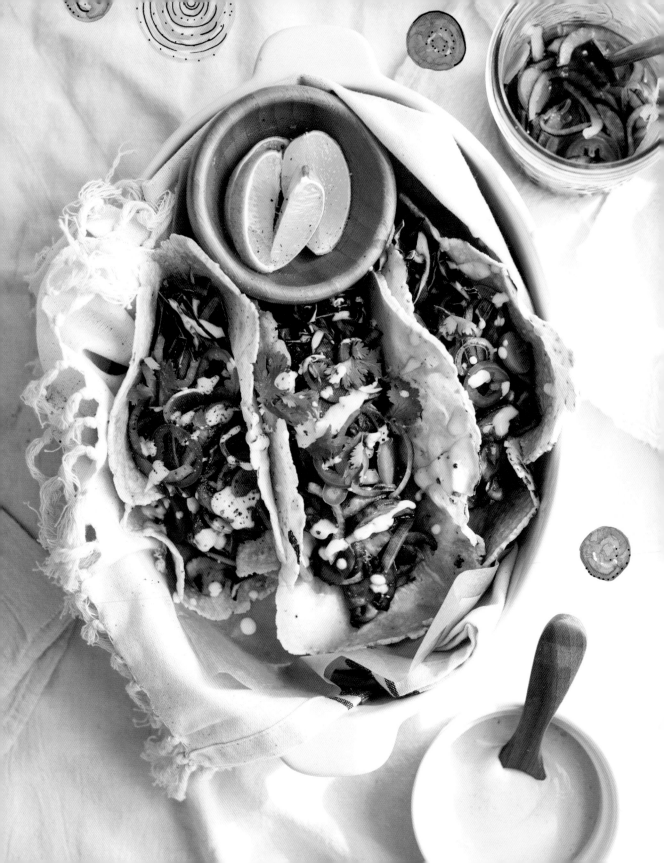

Smoky Mushroom Tacos

There's something magical about the combo of smoky mushrooms, sweet and sour quick pickles, and a kick from Chipotle Cream. Hope these become a part of your weekly menu rotation like they are in my home.

SERVES 2

Quick Pickles

½ cup (120 ml) water

¼ cup (60 ml) apple cider vinegar

1 tablespoon coconut sugar

¼ teaspoon sea salt

½ cup (60 g) thinly sliced red onion

½ large carrot, thinly sliced into rounds

½ jalapeño pepper, ribs removed, seeded, and diced

—

2 teaspoons unrefined coconut oil, grapeseed oil, or avocado oil

3 cups (210 g) sliced cremini and/or button mushrooms

1 shallot, minced

¼ teaspoon liquid smoke (optional, but tasty) or ½ teaspoon smoked paprika

¼ teaspoon sea salt, plus more to taste

Fresh-cracked black pepper (optional)

4 corn tortillas

¼ cup (60 ml) Chipotle Cream (page 28)

1 small lime

Handful shredded cabbage

Handful fresh cilantro

1. To make the Quick Pickles, whisk together the water, vinegar, sugar, and salt until thoroughly dissolved. Fill a mason jar with the onion, carrot, and jalapeño, then pour the vinegar mixture over the top and secure with a lid; give it a good shake. Let it sit at room temperature for at least 1 hour. You can make these two to three weeks in advance; just cover and chill.

2. In a skillet heated to medium, add the oil and sauté the mushrooms, shallot, liquid smoke (if using), salt, and black pepper for 7 to 10 minutes, stirring only occasionally, until the mushrooms start to brown and sear. Try a spoonful and season with more salt if needed. Cover with a lid and set aside.

3. Warm the tortillas in a steamer, on a low gas flame, or in a dry skillet until softened. Layer them on a plate (Tip: A small piece of unbleached parchment layered between keeps them from sticking) and cover with a towel to keep warm as you layer in the fixings.

4. Spoon some mushrooms onto a tortilla and lift some quick pickles from the jar—be sure to drain them—to place on top of the mushrooms. Drizzle with the Chipotle Cream, top with a squeeze of fresh lime, cabbage, and cilantro—repeat until all tacos are filled. Enjoy warm.

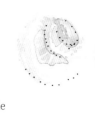

Veggie Enchiladas

If you have the sauce (which you do on page 31), you can
easily riff and make enchiladas. Try collard or kale
wraps instead of tortillas, and fill them with whatever you like.
If you don't have a food processor, break up the cauliflower in
the blender or with elbow grease and a chef's knife—you'll need
1 small head of cauliflower for this recipe.

SERVES 2 TO 4

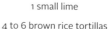

3 cups (315 g) chopped cauliflower (about 1 small head)

2 teaspoons unrefined coconut oil, grapeseed oil, or avocado oil

1 small white onion, diced

½ cup (35 g) broccoli florets, chopped

½ cup (85 g) cooked black beans (roughly ¼ cup/50 g dry; see page 11)

1 cup (145 g) fresh corn kernels

2 garlic cloves, minced

1 tablespoon taco seasoning

2 handfuls fresh cilantro

¼ teaspoon sea salt, plus more to taste

1 small lime

4 to 6 brown rice tortillas

1 batch Enchilada Sauce (page 31)

Half batch Cauliflower Cream (page 32)

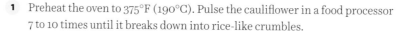

1. Preheat the oven to 375°F (190°C). Pulse the cauliflower in a food processor 7 to 10 times until it breaks down into rice-like crumbles.

2. In a skillet heated to medium, add the oil and sauté the cauliflower "rice," onion, broccoli, and beans for 5 to 7 minutes. Add the corn and garlic and sauté for another 3 minutes. Fold in the taco seasoning, a handful of cilantro, the salt, and a generous squeeze of lime juice. Taste, season with more salt if you like, cover with a lid, and set aside.

3. Warm the tortillas in a steamer, on a low gas flame, or in a dry skillet until softened. Layer them on a plate (unbleached parchment layered between keeps them from sticking) and cover with a towel to keep warm as you fill the enchiladas. Spoon some Enchilada Sauce into an 8 x 12-inch (20 x 30 cm) casserole dish and spread to cover the bottom.

4. Fill one tortilla with a few spoonfuls of seasoned veggies and a spoonful of Cauliflower Cream, and roll up. Place into the casserole dish seam side down. Repeat until all the tortillas are used up and lined side by side in the dish. Cover all with the remaining Enchilada Sauce and drizzle with the remaining Cauliflower Cream. Bake for 25 minutes. Top with the remaining cilantro and a squeeze of lime. Serve warm.

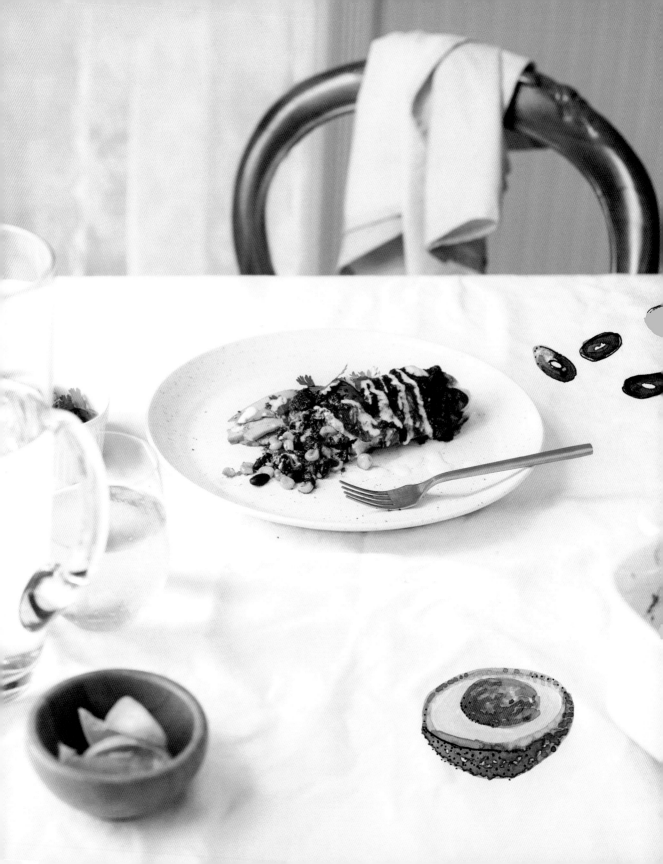

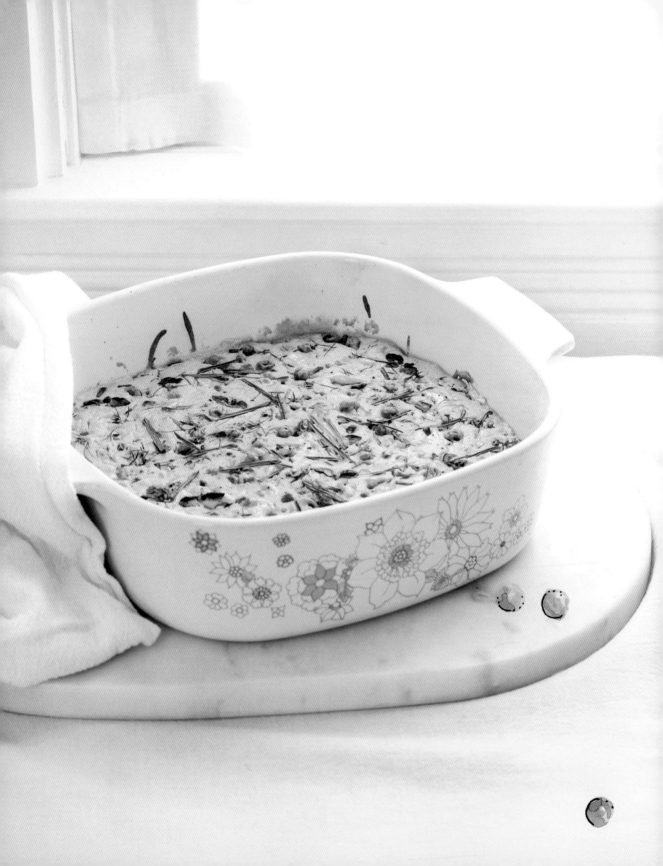

'Banzo Bakes

A bit like the love child of a frittata and farinata flatbread, this comforting quick-bread-style meal is easily transformed from a variety of veggies, herbs, and even leftovers in 30 minutes.

Think about combos you'd use in a Scramble (page 36), or for egg lovers, an omelette, but baked with tasty chickpea flour instead. You can even add eggy flavor by using sulfurous Indian black salt (a.k.a. kala namak) instead of sea salt.

Call it breakfast, lunch, or dinner—it's up to you.

'Banzo Bake combo on this spread: Pea, lemon & spring herbs.

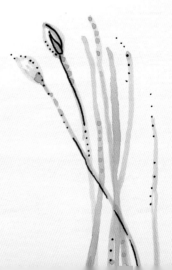

'Banzo Bakes

**6+ SERVINGS
COOK TIME: 25 TO
60 MINUTES**

There are many ways to prepare a 'Banzo Bake. Use eight to ten 3- to 5-inch (7.5 to 12.5 cm) ramekins for single servings or an 8- to 10-inch (20 to 25 cm) cast-iron skillet or baking dish for sliceable servings. In Step 3, make sure the Cream is thick but pourable, so if needed, blend 1 tablespoon of water at a time into the Cream until you reach this consistency. You are also using only a half batch of the Cream, so save the rest for Tacos (page 217) or Sriracha Mac (page 188).

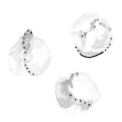

What you need no matter what:

¼ cup (60 ml) unrefined coconut oil, grapeseed oil, or avocado oil, plus more for cooking

2 cups (220 g) garbanzo bean flour

2½ cups (600 ml) hot water, or more if needed

1 teaspoon plus a pinch sea salt

1 to 3 garlic cloves (optional), minced

1 to 2 teaspoons fresh lemon juice (optional)

Fresh-cracked black pepper (optional)

1 Preheat the oven to 375°F (190°C) and grease the baking dish(es) you want to use with **oil.** If you have a cast-iron skillet, use that for sautéing and baking—it'll be a one-pot meal. But first, make a Garbanzo Base mixture by whisking together the **garbanzo bean flour** with 1 cup of the Cream, **2½ cups (600 ml) hot water**, **¼ cup (60 ml) oil**, and **1 teaspoon salt** until combined. Set aside.

Cream   Choose one or combine

1¼ cups (300 ml) Cashew Cream (half batch from page 32)

1½ cups (335 g) Coconut Yogurt (half batch from page 94, prepare 1 to 5 days in advance) or store-bought plain nondairy yogurt

2 In a skillet heated to medium, add 1 tablespoon **oil** and sauté Dense Veggies (if using) for 15 to 20 minutes, until easily pierced with a fork, but firm. Add Sauté Veggies (if using) to the skillet; cook over medium heat for 5 to 7 minutes, until softened. Add the **garlic** if you like and sauté for 3 more minutes. Squeeze the **lemon juice** (if using) over all. Evenly distribute the veggies in the baking dish(es)—unless they're staying in the cast-iron skillet.

Dense Veggies

½ TO 1 CUP TOTAL

Choose one or combine, or skip altogether

Sweet potatoes   Potatoes

Winter squash   Carrots

Beets

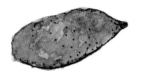

Sauté Veggies

Choose one or combine, or skip altogether

½ to 1 cup (70 to 135 g) chopped asparagus

1 small onion or 1 large shallot, diced

1 red, yellow, or orange bell pepper, seeded, ribs removed, and diced

½ to 2 cups (55 to 215 g) chopped cauliflower

½ to 2 cups (35 to 140 g) sliced mushrooms

1 to 3 cups (30 to 90 g) chopped hearty greens

½ to 1 cup (50 to 100 g) diced celery

½ to 2 cups (45 to 180 g) chopped broccoli

3 Give your Garbanzo Base & Cream mixture a whisking and pour into the baking dish(es) over the veggies, then drizzle with the remaining Cream. Evenly distribute Raw Veggies and Extras (if using) into the dish(es) or skillet and swirl in Sauce (if using). Sprinkle the top(s) with a pinch of **salt,** more herbs if you like, and/or **black pepper** (if using). Bake ramekins for 25 to 30 minutes, until firm, or a skillet or baking dishes for 40 to 60 minutes. For extra browning, broil for 2 to 3 more minutes after baking. Cool for 10 minutes to set; serve warm.

Raw Veggies

Choose one or combine, or skip altogether

½ to 2 cups (90 to 360 g) seeded, diced tomatoes

½ to 2 cups (55 to 225 g) sliced summer squash

½ to 2 cups (70 to 290 g) green peas

Extras

¼ TO 1 CUP

Choose one or combine, or skip altogether

Marinated goods (pitted olives, artichoke hearts)

Fresh herbs

Pine nuts

Raisins

Sun-dried tomatoes

Sauce

Choose one or combine, or skip altogether

¼ to ½ cup (60 to 120 ml) Chimichurri (page 30)

¼ to ½ cup (60 to 120 ml) Supergreen Pesto (page 33)

1 to 3 tablespoons harissa (jar)

¼ to ½ cup (65 to 130 g) salsa

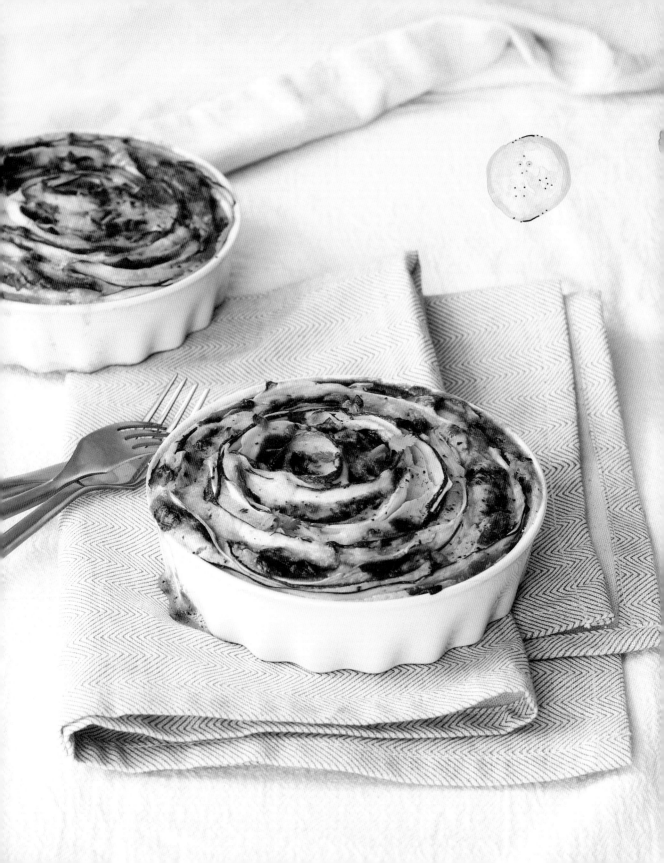

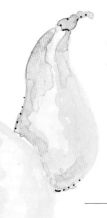

Harissa Swirl 'Banzo Bake

If you have one, use a mandoline for paper-thin veggie ribbons, but a chef's knife works fine. You can also use diced veggies instead. You only need a half batch of Cashew Cream for this recipe—save the rest for Mmmaki (page 205)!

SERVES 4+

2½ cups (600 ml) hot water, plus more for Cashew Cream if needed

1¼ cups (300 ml) Cashew Cream (page 32)

1 medium yellow squash, sliced into ribbons lengthwise

1 medium zucchini, sliced into ribbons lengthwise

Pinch plus 1 teaspoon sea salt, plus more to taste

2 cups (220 g) garbanzo bean flour

¼ cup (60 ml) unrefined coconut oil, grapeseed oil, or avocado oil, plus more for cooking

1 large shallot, sliced into thin rounds

2 to 3 garlic cloves, minced

2 teaspoons fresh lemon juice

¼ cup (5 g) fresh cilantro

¼ cup (15 g) fresh parsley

3 tablespoons harissa (jar)

Fresh-cracked black pepper

1. Whisk or blend 1 tablespoon water at a time into the Cashew Cream if it's not already a pourable consistency—you want it like melted ice cream.

2. Preheat the oven to 375°F (190°C). Lay the squash and zucchini ribbons on a kitchen towel; sprinkle with the pinch of salt and let them rest for 10 minutes. Lay another dish towel on top of them and press out water.

3. Whisk together the garbanzo bean flour with the hot water, 1 cup (240 ml) of the Cashew Cream, ¼ cup (60 ml) of the oil, and 1 teaspoon salt until combined. Set aside. In an 8- to 10-inch (20 to 25 cm) skillet heated to medium, add 1 tablespoon oil and sauté the shallot for 5 minutes, until it starts to brown. Add the garlic and stir together for another 3 minutes. Drizzle with the lemon juice; transfer to a small bowl.

4. Arrange the squash and zucchini ribbons in a swirl directly in the skillet, or in 3- to 6-inch (8 to 15 cm) ramekins or an 8- to 10-inch (20 to 25 cm) ceramic baking dish with the shallot and garlic. Sprinkle half of the herbs on top and pour the garbanzo base over and between the squash, filling the baking vessel(s). Drizzle with the harissa and remaining Cashew Cream. Sprinkle with the remaining herbs, a few grinds of pepper, and salt to taste.

5. For a skillet or baking dish, bake for 40 to 60 minutes—for ramekins, bake for 25 to 30 minutes, until firm. For extra browning, broil for 2 to 3 more minutes after baking. Cool for 10 minutes to set; serve warm.

Rainbow Chard & Golden Raisin 'Banzo Bake

A delicious combination of sautéed onion, sweet raisins, and loads of gorgeous chard. Serve it topped with homemade Coconut Yogurt (page 94), paired with fresh herb salad, or drizzled with balsamic vinaigrette. If you don't have a cast-iron skillet, use a ceramic baking dish or ramekins (note important baking time differences in Step 3 on page 229). Make a full batch of Coconut Yogurt—you only need half for this recipe—and use the rest for a Maple-Spiced Pear & Toasted Pecan Parfait (page 99)!

SERVES 6+

2½ cups (600 ml) hot water, plus more for Coconut Yogurt if needed

1½ cups (335 g) unsweetened Coconut Yogurt (page 94), or any store-bought plain nondairy yogurt

2 cups (220 g) garbanzo bean flour

¼ cup (60 ml) unrefined coconut oil, grapeseed oil, or avocado oil, plus more for cooking

1 teaspoon sea salt, plus more to taste

1 small yellow onion, sliced

3 packed cups (105 g) chopped chard

2 teaspoons fresh lemon juice

¼ cup (40 g) golden raisins

1 tablespoon fresh chives, plus more if you like

2 teaspoons fresh thyme, plus more if you like

Fresh-cracked black pepper

1. Preheat the oven to 375°F (190°C). Whisk or blend 1 tablespoon water at a time into the yogurt if it's not already a pourable consistency—you want it like melted ice cream. Whisk together the garbanzo bean flour with the hot water, 1 cup (225 g) of the yogurt, the oil, and salt until combined. Set aside so the batter can rest.

2. In an 8- to 10-inch (20 to 25 cm) cast-iron skillet heated to medium, add 1 tablespoon oil and sauté the onion for 5 to 7 minutes, until it starts to brown. Add the chard and sauté for 3 minutes, or until it begins to wilt. Remove from the heat. Drizzle with the lemon juice and evenly sprinkle with raisins, chives, and thyme. Then pour the garbanzo-yogurt mixture over the contents of the skillet, give it a quick stir, and drizzle with the remaining yogurt. Sprinkle with salt to taste, a few grinds of pepper, extra herbs if you like, and place in the oven to bake for 40 minutes, or until the top and edges are firm. For extra browning, broil for 2 to 3 more minutes. Cool for 10 minutes so the bake sets—serve warm.

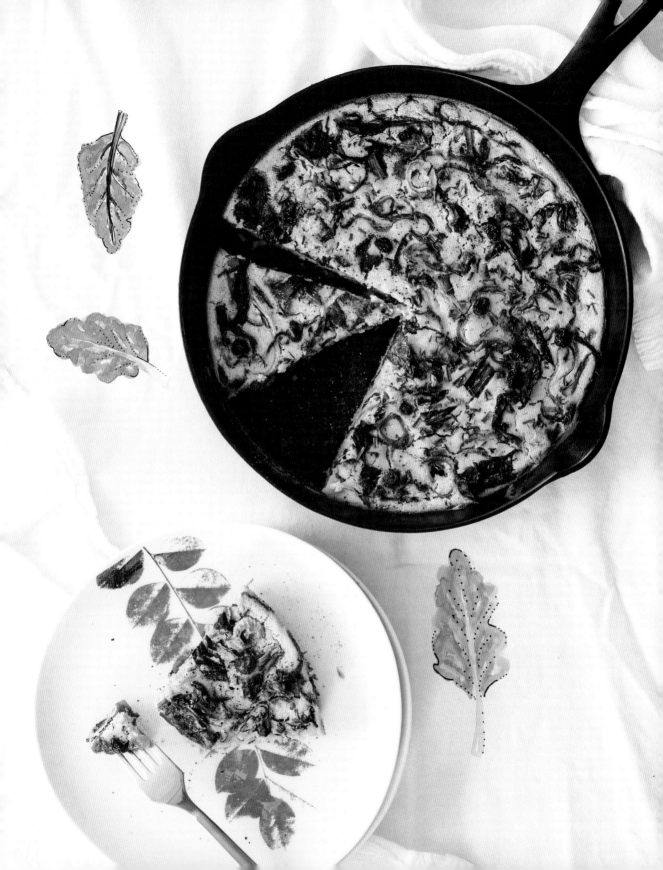

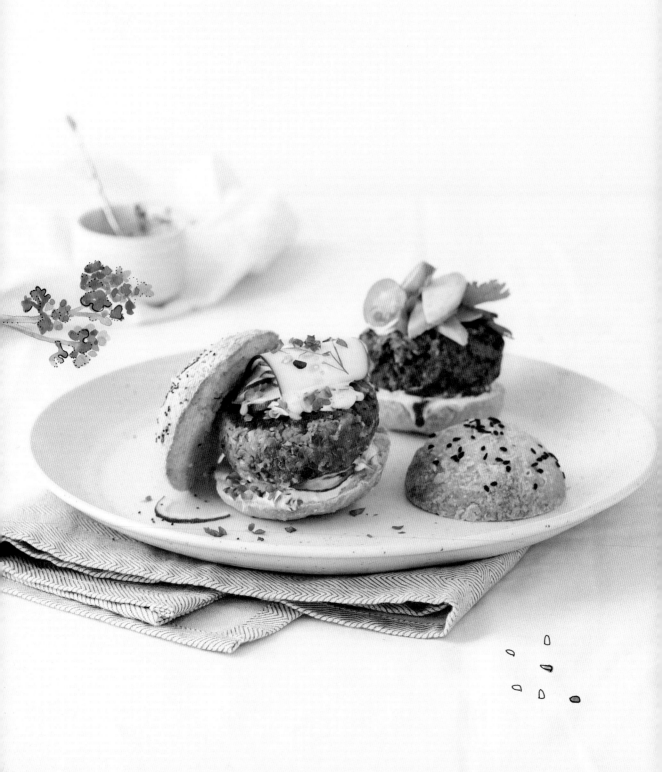

Learn how to make gluten-free slider buns:
glutenfreebakingacademy.com

Veggie Burgers

Move over, gray cardboard patties—there are a million and one ways to make crave-worthy veggie burgers and sliders with this template.

Make a batch or three and freeze to reheat for future meals. Fry them up with taco seasoning and crumble for "taco meat." Add them to salads for texture. Fold them with Italian herbs and spices to make a "meaty" tomato sauce. You can even roll them into not-meatballs for spaghetti or subs.

Veggie Burger combos on this spread:
Chickpea-potato-cauliflower slider; Black Bean Slider (page 238);
Italian-Style Lentil & Mushroom (Not)Meatball Slider (page 241).

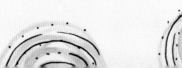
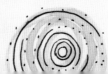

Veggie Burgers

The game-changer ingredient here is psyllium—no more dry, sad veggie burger crumbles with each bite. It binds like a champ, holds moisture, and adds fiber. If using a salted seasoning mix in Step 3, skip the salt called for and, after seasoning, add more to taste.

MAKES 8 BURGERS
COOK TIME: 20 TO 35 MINUTES

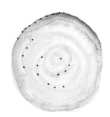

What you need no matter what:

2 tablespoons unrefined coconut or grapeseed oil

1 cup (160 g) diced onion (any kind) or shallot

2 to 5 garlic cloves (optional), minced

2 tablespoons water

1 teaspoons sea salt, plus more to taste

1 In a skillet heated to medium, add 1 tablespoon **oil** and sauté Dense Veggies for 10 to 20 minutes, until easily pierced with a fork but firm, not mushy.

Dense Veggies

2 CUPS DICED TOTAL

Choose one or combine

Sweet potatoes

Winter squash (remove skin and seeds)

Beets

Potatoes (any kind)

Carrots

2 Add the **onion or shallot** and Veggies to skillet—sauté for 5 minutes, or until softened. Add the **garlic** if you like and sauté for 1 to 2 more minutes. Add Protein and stir together for 2 more minutes. Transfer to a food processor but don't pulse yet.

Veggies -------- *and* --------> Protein

Choose one or combine

½ to 1 cup (75 to 150 g) diced bell pepper (any kind)

½ cup (50 g) diced celery

1 cup (90 g) diced broccoli

½ to 1 cup chopped hearty greens (kale, chard, spinach)

1 cup (105 g) diced cauliflower

½ to 1 cup (70 to 145 g) green peas

1 to 2 cups (70 to 140 g) sliced mushrooms (any kind)

1 cup (110 g) sliced summer squash (any kind)

2 CUPS TOTAL

Choose one or combine, page 11 for cooking tips

Oats, uncooked

Precook all of the following:

Beans (any kind)

Buckwheat, hulled

Chickpeas

Lentils

Millet

Quinoa

3 Chop and add Fresh (if using) to the food processor. Sprinkle Binder evenly over all and add the **water**, the **salt**, and Flavor (if using). Pulse together 20 to 30 times, until just broken up with texture and bits of color intact. Season with more salt or Flavor if needed. Stir to incorporate.

Fresh

Choose one or combine, or skip altogether

2 to 4 tablespoons chopped fresh herbs (sage, thyme, basil, cilantro, rosemary, dill, chives, oregano)

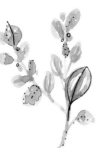

Binder

Choose one

2½ teaspoons whole psyllium husk

2 teaspoons ground psyllium husk

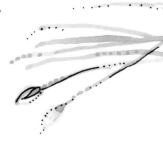

Flavor

Choose one or combine, or skip altogether

*Choose any of these in combination **OR*** - - - - - - - - - - - - - - - - - - - → *Choose one of these by itself*

2 to 4 teaspoons nutritional yeast	¼ teaspoon cayenne pepper	¼ to 1 teaspoon liquid smoke	1 to 4 teaspoons Italian seasoning
¼ to ½ teaspoon chipotle powder	1 teaspoon grated citrus zest	¼ to ½ cup (60 to 120 g) sun-dried tomatoes	1 to 4 teaspoons taco seasoning
1 to 2 teaspoons Sriracha	1 to 4 teaspoons fresh citrus juice	1 to 3 teaspoons vegan Worcestershire	1 to 4 teaspoons Montreal steak seasoning
1 to 4 teaspoons coconut aminos	1 to 2 tablespoons minced jalapeño	½ to 1 teaspoon fresh-cracked black pepper	1 to 4 teaspoons garam masala
1 to 2 tablespoons Dijon or whole-grain mustard	½ to 2 teaspoons smoked paprika	1 to 4 teaspoons rough-chopped fennel seed	1 to 2 tablespoons harissa (jar)
½ to 1 teaspoon red pepper flakes	1 to 2 teaspoons coconut aminos, soy sauce, or tamari		1 to 4 teaspoons miso (any kind)

4 Form patties with your hands—heat a skillet to medium-low, adding 1 tablespoon oil. Slow-cook the patties for 10 to 15 minutes on each side, until browned—you'll only need to flip once, maybe twice—let them cook! Serve warm.

Black Bean Sliders

Serve these tasty sliders with Smoky BBQ Sauce (page 30), Chipotle Cream (page 28), and sliced avocado. They're a perfect balance of hearty, spicy, and creamy-cool for a dinner at home or for party food you can feel good about.

MAKES 10 TO 12 SLIDERS OR 5 TO 6 FULL-SIZE BURGERS

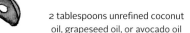

2 tablespoons unrefined coconut oil, grapeseed oil, or avocado oil

2 cups (265 g) diced sweet potato

1 cup (150 g) diced red bell pepper

1 cup (160 g) diced yellow onion

5 garlic cloves, minced

1½ cups (255 g) cooked black beans (roughly ½ cup/95 g dry; see page 11)

½ cup (40 g) rolled oats

½ cup (10 g) chopped fresh cilantro

2 tablespoons taco seasoning

2 tablespoons water

1 tablespoon nutritional yeast (optional)

2 teaspoons fresh lime juice

2 teaspoons ground psyllium husk

1 teaspoon grated lime zest

1 teaspoon sea salt, plus more to taste

½ teaspoon fresh-cracked black pepper

Gluten-free, egg-free slider buns (optional)

1. In a skillet heated to medium, add 1 tablespoon of the oil and sauté the sweet potato for 10 to 20 minutes, until easily pierced with a fork, but firm, not mushy.

2. Add the bell pepper and onion and sauté over medium heat for 5 to 10 minutes, until softened and browning a bit. Add the garlic and sauté for 2 to 3 minutes. Transfer to a food processor with the black beans and oats. Add the cilantro, taco seasoning, water, nutritional yeast, lime juice, psyllium, lime zest, salt, and black pepper. Pulse together 20 to 25 times, until just broken up and sticky with texture and bits of color intact. Taste— if needed, season with more salt or seasonings. Pulse or stir to incorporate.

3. Form 2- to 3-inch (5 to 7.5 cm) patties with your hands. Heat a skillet to medium-low; add the remaining oil. Slow-cook the patties for 10 to 15 minutes on each side, until browned—you'll only need to flip once, maybe twice—let them cook! Serve warm.

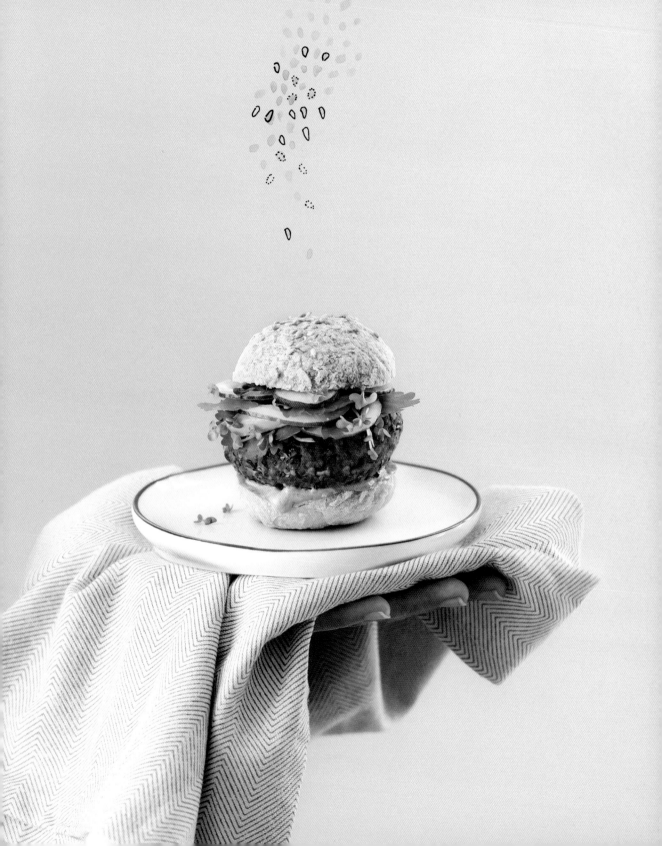

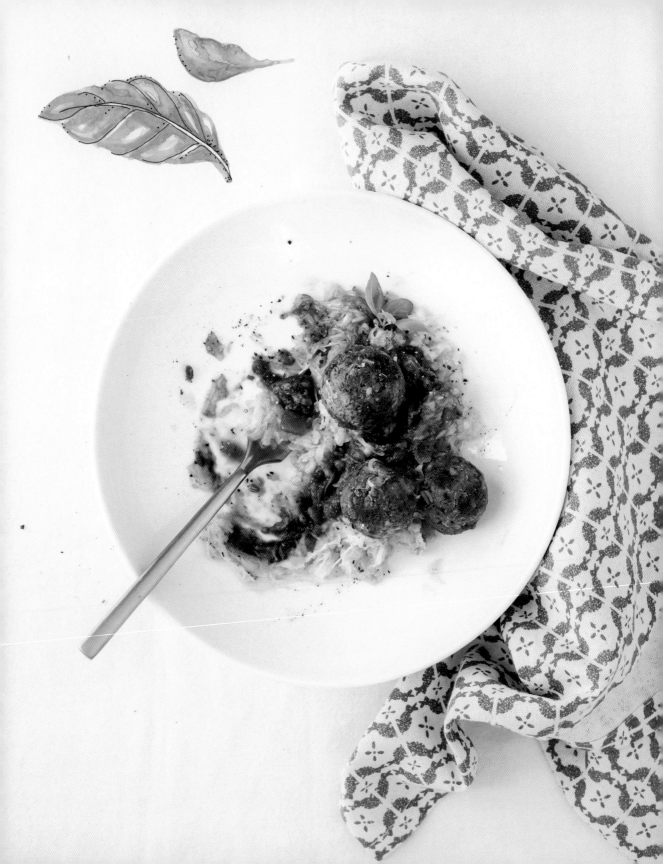

Italian-Style Lentil & Mushroom (Not)Meatballs

Try these (not)meatballs nestled in a sub roll, served as an appetizer with a delicious dipping sauce (pages 28–33), or with roasted spaghetti squash and Maudie's Tomato Sauce (page 32) for a pasta-free spaghetti and (not)meatballs that's sooo good. You can shape them into burgers or sliders, too!

MAKES 20 TO 24 MEATBALLS OR 5 TO 6 FULL-SIZED BURGERS

2 tablespoons unrefined coconut oil, grapeseed oil, or avocado oil

2 cups (260 g) diced carrots

1 cup (70 g) chopped portobello mushrooms

1 cup (160 g) diced yellow onion

2 cups (400 g) cooked green, brown, or French green lentils (roughly ¾ cup/140 g dry; see page 11)

2 tablespoons water

1 tablespoon chopped fresh basil

1 tablespoon chopped fresh parsley

1 tablespoon chopped fresh oregano

1 tablespoon chopped fresh thyme

3 garlic cloves, minced

2 teaspoons ground psyllium husk

2 teaspoons rough-chopped fennel seed

1 teaspoon fresh-cracked black pepper

1 teaspoon sea salt, plus more to taste

½ teaspoon red pepper flakes

½ teaspoon smoked paprika

1. In a skillet heated to medium, add 1 tablespoon of the oil and sauté the carrots for 20 minutes, until easily pierced with a fork but firm, not mushy.

2. Add the mushrooms and onion and sauté over medium heat for 5 to 10 minutes, until softened and browning a bit. Transfer to a food processor with the remaining ingredients. Pulse together 30 to 35 times, until just broken up and sticky with texture and bits of color intact. Taste—if needed, season with more salt or seasonings. Pulse or stir to incorporate.

3. Form 1½-inch (4 cm) meatballs with your hands. Heat a skillet to medium and add the remaining oil. Slow-cook the meatballs, rotating often, for 10 to 15 minutes, until browned on all sides. Serve warm.

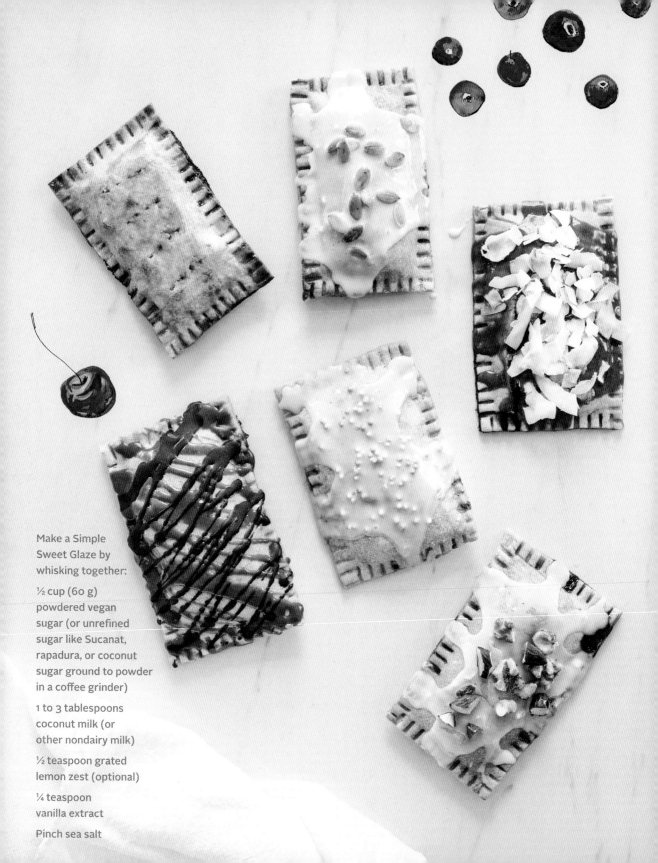

Make a Simple
Sweet Glaze by
whisking together:

½ cup (60 g)
powdered vegan
sugar (or unrefined
sugar like Sucanat,
rapadura, or coconut
sugar ground to powder
in a coffee grinder)

1 to 3 tablespoons
coconut milk (or
other nondairy milk)

½ teaspoon grated
lemon zest (optional)

¼ teaspoon
vanilla extract

Pinch sea salt

Hand Pies

A smidge labor intensive (glass-half-empty people) or meditative (glass-half-full people), but truly worth it, these pies are a great way to use up leftovers to create something special. Try Taco filling (page 217) or Scrambles (page 36), chopped veggies, cooked grains, legumes and/or beans tossed with salsa, Chimichurri (page 30), Enchilada Sauce (page 31), or even Smoky BBQ Sauce (page 30) for savory mini pie filling.

For sweet pies, try Compote (page 90) or fresh fruit (frozen works, too) tossed with jam and/or Probiotic Cream Cheese (page 128) or Cashew Cream (page 32).

In the spirit of keeping it real, these filling ideas are simple—know that if a filling would taste good on its own, it'll taste good inside a crust!

Don't forget to dip them into tasty sauces (page 28)—have fun!

Hand Pie Combos on this spread left to right, top to bottom:
Mixed berry with maple glaze; cranberry-apple-cardamom with vanilla glaze & pepitas; strawberry, toasted coconut & sucanat glaze; bing cherry, coconut sugar glaze & dark chocolate; spiced pear compote, vanilla glaze; raspberry, Meyer lemon glaze & toasted nuts.

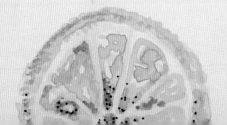

Hand Pies

**MAKES 10+ 6-INCH (15 CM) PIES
OR 20+ 3-INCH (7.5 CM) PIES
COOK TIME: 15 TO 30 MINUTES**

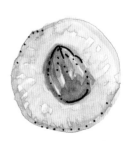
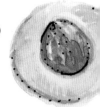

Flour-to-water ratio can vary based on the type of flour, the season, even the humidity in your home; start with less water, adding more until you get a moist-not-sticky ball of dough. Find the sweet spot: Roll and shape dough in floured palms. Too dry? Wet your hands and press moisture into the dough. Too wet? Dust with flour and work it in. Bean flours (best with savory fillings) tend to be sticky and want less water, while absorbent flours like oat want more. As you work, drape a damp towel over unused dough to keep it from drying out.

What you need no matter what:

A few pinches plus 1 teaspoon sea salt

½ to 1 cup (120 to 240 ml) warm water, plus more if needed

Maple syrup for glazing (optional)

1 Preheat the oven to 400°F (200°C). Pull three cookie-sheet-sized pieces of unbleached parchment paper; use one to line a baking sheet and set the others aside for rolling dough. For a savory hand pie, in a large bowl, fold together Filling, Sauce, Oil 1, and Cream (if using), and a pinch of **salt** if needed; set aside. For a sweet pie, skip to Step 2.

Filling ···· *and* ···▶ Sauce ······ *and* ···▶ Oil 1

3 TO 4 CUPS TOTAL
Choose one or combine, or skip altogether

Scramble (page 36)

Veggie Burgers
(page 235)

Bites & Tots
(page 159)

Hearty greens
(page 26)

Taco filling
(page 217)

Sautéed or
roasted veggies

Cooked grains

Cooked legumes
and beans

¼ TO ½ CUP (60 TO 120 ML) TOTAL
Choose one or skip altogether

Supergreen Pesto
(page 33)

Chimichurri
(page 30)

Salsa

Smoky BBQ Sauce
(page 30)

Enchilada Sauce
(page 31)

Maudie's Tomato
Sauce (page 32)

**3 TABLESPOONS
TOTAL**
Choose one

Unrefined coconut oil

Grapeseed oil

Cream

¼ TO ½ CUP (60 TO 120 ML) TOTAL
Choose one or skip altogether

Probiotic
Cream Cheese
(page 128)

Cashew Cream
(page 32)

Cauliflower Cream
(page 32)

Chipotle Cream
(page 28)

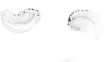

2   Sweet pie only: If using compote, strain the liquid from the fruit and save it for Nice Cream (page 279) or Coconut Yogurt (page 94)—you'll use the fruit for filling. In a bowl, combine Sweet Filling, Stickiness, a pinch of **salt**, and Special Additions (if using); set aside.

Sweet Filling ······ *and* ·····→ Stickiness

2 CUPS TOTAL
Choose one
or combine

Pome fruit, cored
and diced

Stone fruit, pitted
and chopped

Berries

Tropical fruit,
chopped

1 CUP TOTAL
Choose one
or combine

Compote & Fruit
Butter (page 90)

Fruit jam or jelly

Special Additions

Choose one or combine,
or skip altogether

¼ cup (40 g) dried
fruit (raisins, dates,
cherries)

1 to 2 teaspoons
grated citrus zest

¼ cup (60 g)
Probiotic Cream
Cheese (page 128)

¼ cup (60 ml)
Cashew Cream
(page 32)

---

3   In a food processor (or using elbow grease), mix together Flours, Binder, and 1 teaspoon **salt**. Add Oil 2 until crumbly. Add the **water**—adding 1 tablespoon more at a time if needed, until a moist but non-sticky dough ball forms. Flour your hands to roll the dough into a ball and place on a sheet of parchment. Place another sheet of parchment on top; press and use a rolling pin to flatten to ⅛ inch (3 mm). Dust with flour as you work.

Flours ···· *and* ···→ Binder ···· *and* ···→ Oil 2

2½ CUPS TOTAL
Choose one or combine

Garbanzo bean flour

Oat flour

Gluten-free
all-purpose

Choose one

1 teaspoon whole
psyllium husk

½ teaspoon ground
psyllium husk

**¼ CUP (60 ML)
TOTAL**
Choose one

Unrefined coconut oil

Grapeseed oil

---

4   Use a knife and small bowl, or a pizza cutter, to cut 3- or 6-inch (7.5 to 15 cm) round or square pieces of dough. Transfer half of the small pieces or all of the large pieces to the lined baking sheet. Spoon filling onto the centers of the pieces, only on one half of the large pieces or the entire centers of the small pieces, leaving ¾ inch (2 cm) unfilled around the edges. Using a finger dipped in water, trace the edges of the crust. Fold the dough of the large pieces over the filling, or top the small pieces with another piece of dough so the edges meet. Press the edges together gently with a fork. Make sure the pies are 1 inch (2.5 cm) apart. For a simple glaze, paint the tops with **maple syrup,** even on the savory pies. Bake for 20 minutes, until dry and browning.

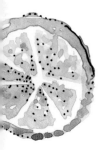

Millet & Veggie Empanadas

Dip these into Chimichurri (page 30), fresh salsa,
Enchilada Sauce (page 31), or Chipotle Cream (page 28).

MAKES 8 TO 10

¼ cup (60 ml) plus 3 tablespoons unrefined coconut oil, grapeseed oil, or avocado oil

½ cup (65 g) diced sweet potato

½ cup (75 g) diced red bell pepper

½ cup (80 g) diced yellow onion

1 cup (170 g) cooked black beans (roughly ⅓ cup/65 g dry; see page 11)

1 cup (175 g) cooked millet (roughly 1/3 cup/65 g dry; see page 11)

¼ cup (15 g) chopped fresh cilantro

2 garlic cloves, minced

1 tablespoon taco seasoning

1 teaspoon grated lime zest

1 teaspoon fresh lime juice

½ teaspoon ground cinnamon

1½ teaspoons sea salt, plus more to taste

2½ cups (275 g) garbanzo bean flour, plus more for rolling

½ teaspoon ground psyllium husk

½ cup (120 ml) warm water, plus more if needed

Maple syrup (optional for glazing)

1. In a skillet heated to medium-high, add 1 tablespoon of the oil and sauté the sweet potato for 10 to 20 minutes, until easily pierced with a fork but firm, not mushy. Add the pepper and onion and sauté for 7 to 10 minutes, until softened and starting to brown. Add the beans, millet, cilantro, garlic, taco seasoning, lime zest, lime juice, cinnamon, and ½ teaspoon of the salt, or more to taste. Stir together for 3 minutes, remove from the heat, and stir in 2 more tablespoons of the oil; set aside.

2. Preheat the oven to 400°F (200°C) and line a baking sheet with unbleached parchment paper. In a food processor, pulse together the flour, psyllium, and 1 teaspoon of the salt; add the remaining ¼ cup (60 ml) oil and pulse until crumbly. Add the water plus 1 tablespoon more at a time if needed, until a moist but non-sticky dough ball forms. Flour your hands, roll the dough into a ball, and place on a sheet of parchment paper. Dust with flour; top with another sheet of parchment. Use a rolling pin to flatten the dough to ⅛ inch (3 mm) thick. Peel back the top sheet; dust with flour.

3. Use a 6-inch (15 cm) round cookie cutter or cereal bowl to cut out crusts. Transfer to the baking sheet and spoon filling onto half of a crust, leaving ¾ inch (2 cm) unfilled around the edges. Trace the edge of the crust with water. Fold the crust over and press the edges together with a fork. Repeat until all empanadas are formed; arrange them 1 inch (2.5 cm) apart. Brush the tops with maple syrup (if using); bake for 20 minutes, until browned.

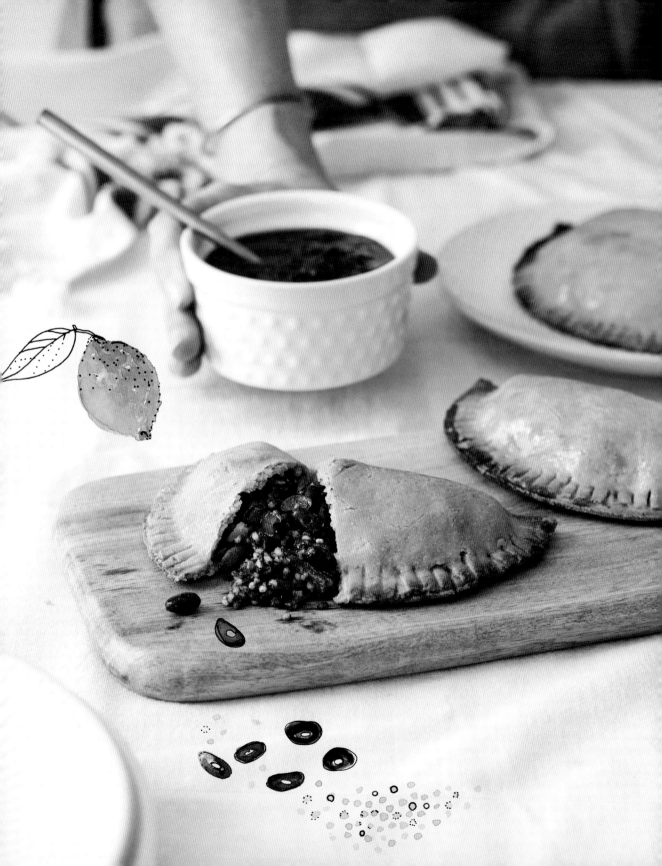

Strawberry-Oat Hand Pies

Split the amounts in half if you only want 8 to 12 pies. I call for
3- to 4-inch (7.5 to 10 cm) round cookie cutters, but you can use a knife
to create any shape. To effortlessly work with rolled-out dough,
slide it (and the parchment) onto a cutting board and freeze for a few
minutes to harden. Then, easily transfer from surface to surface.

MAKES 16 TO 24

Strawberry Compote
(based on page 90)

2 pounds (1 kg) strawberries,
tops removed and chopped

1 teaspoon grated lemon zest

2 teaspoons fresh lemon juice

½ cup (120 ml) raw,
unpasteurized honey

—

1½ teaspoons vanilla extract

½ cup (120 ml) water

Pinch sea salt

½ cup (75 g) strawberries,
chopped into tiny pieces

2 cups (210 g) oat flour,
plus more for rolling

½ cup (75 g) gluten-free
all-purpose flour (a non-bean
flour mix)

1 teaspoon sea salt

½ teaspoon ground psyllium husk

¼ cup (60 ml) unrefined
coconut oil

½ cup (120 ml) warm water,
plus more if needed

Maple syrup
(optional for glazing)

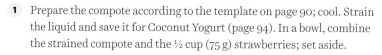

1. Prepare the compote according to the template on page 90; cool. Strain
   the liquid and save it for Coconut Yogurt (page 94). In a bowl, combine
   the strained compote and the ½ cup (75 g) strawberries; set aside.

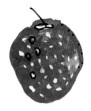

2. Preheat the oven to 400°F (200°C) and line two baking sheets with
   unbleached parchment paper. In a food processor, pulse together the flours,
   salt, and psyllium until well mixed. Add the oil and pulse until crumbly.
   Add the water, plus 1 tablespoon more at a time if needed, until a moist but
   non-sticky dough ball forms. Flour your hands, roll the dough into a ball,
   and place on a sheet of parchment paper. Dust with flour and place another
   sheet of parchment on top. Use a rolling pin to flatten the dough to about
   ⅛ inch (3 mm) thick. Peel back the top sheet and dust with flour.

3. Use a 3- to 4-inch (7.5 to 10 cm) round cookie cutter to cut out crusts. Use an
   offset spatula or large knife to lift and transfer half to the baking sheets,
   arranging them 1 inch (2.5 cm) apart. Spoon filling into the center of each
   crust, leaving ¾ inch (2 cm) unfilled around the edges. Trace the edge of a
   crust with water. Lay another crust on top and press the edges together
   with a fork. Repeat until all pies are formed. Brush the tops with maple
   syrup (if using) and bake for 20 minutes, until browned and bubbling.

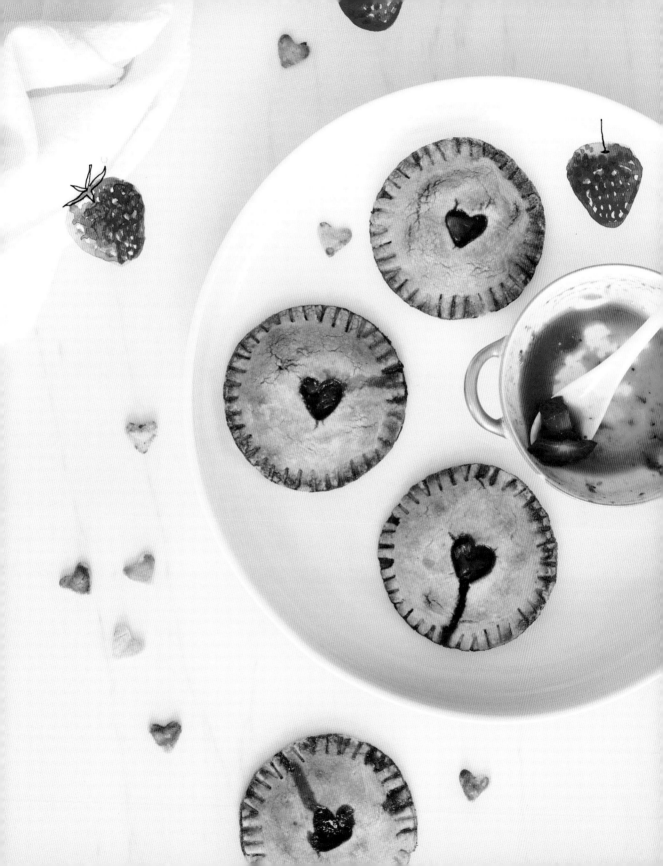

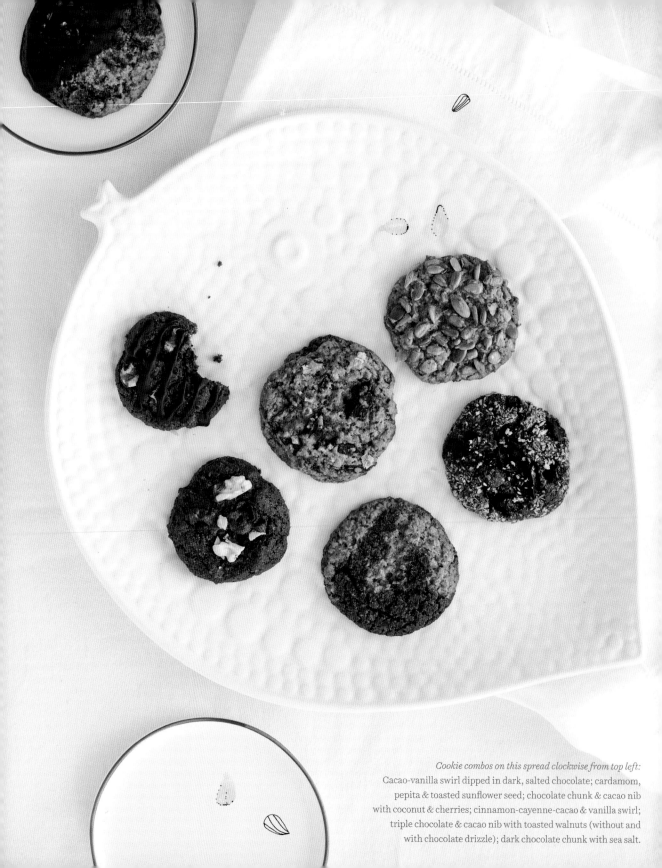

Cookie combos on this spread clockwise from top left:
Cacao-vanilla swirl dipped in dark, salted chocolate; cardamom,
pepita & toasted sunflower seed; chocolate chunk & cacao nib
with coconut & cherries; cinnamon-cayenne-cacao & vanilla swirl;
triple chocolate & cacao nib with toasted walnuts (without and
with chocolate drizzle); dark chocolate chunk with sea salt.

Sweet Tooth

I GREW UP EATING PACKAGED HAND PIES and ice cream sundaes drowned in butterscotch. Being the first grandchild of many, I used to scale my grandmother's cabinets to reach the mile-long row of cookie jars that lined the length of her counter, only to venture further upward to the holy grail "candy cabinet" to share the spoils with giddy, bouncing cousins and little brother below. I can still hear the angels singing as I opened the door to the candy bars, the "fancy" cookies, and all the other treats that turn a kid's eyes into swirling starlight mints. Me and sugar have been frenemies for my whole life, and while I've made incredible strides to get off the sugar IV drip, sometimes you just want a treat.

Is it such a tall order to ask for a goodie that looks and tastes delicious without compromising your goals, or making you feel terrible afterwards? No. It. Is. Not.

Ask and you shall receive, my loves. Creamy ice cream, chewy cookies, and nostalgic treats can be yours if you just turn the page. Cue the twinkly, magical music. . . .

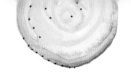

Cookies

16 TO 18 COOKIES
BAKE TIME: 20 TO 25 MINUTES

The main base here is almond flour, but if you're nut-free, substitute with equal amounts of gluten-free all-purpose flour, or a combo of oat, sorghum, and brown rice flour. Also, arrowroot provides a nice crumb, but you can skip it. Pretoast Fold-Ins like coconut, nuts, and seeds before adding to the dough for extra flavor. Applesauce is a great go-to Purée to keep in the fridge. And note that this cookie dough (or baked cookies) can be folded into some Nice Cream (page 279). Just sayin'.

What you need no matter what:

½ cup plus 2 tablespoons (70 g) blanched almond flour

1 tablespoon arrowroot starch/flour

1 teaspoon baking powder

½ teaspoon sea salt

3 tablespoons warm water

2 tablespoons unrefined coconut oil, gently warmed to liquid

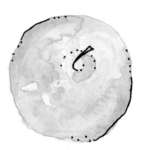

1 Preheat the oven to 350°F (180°C); line a baking sheet with unbleached parchment paper or a silicone baking mat. In a large bowl, sift together Sweet, Flour, the **almond flour, arrowroot, baking powder, salt,** and Spice (if using).

Sweet ----- *and* ----> Flour

¾ CUP (150 G) TOTAL
Choose one or combine

Sucanat

Rapadura

Coconut sugar

½ CUP TOTAL
Choose one or combine

Brown rice flour

Oat flour

Sorghum flour

Gluten-free all-purpose flour

Teff flour

Millet flour

Buckwheat flour

Spice

Choose one or combine, or skip altogether

1 to 2 teaspoons ground cinnamon

Pinch to ¼ teaspoon cayenne pepper

Pinch to ¼ teaspoon ground cardamom

2 to 3 tablespoons cocoa/cacao powder

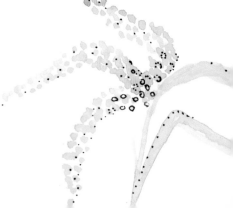

2 In another large bowl, whisk together Purée, Acid, and Flavor (if using) with the **water** and warm **oil** until thoroughly combined.

Purée ------- *and* -------→ Acid

¼ CUP TOTAL

Choose one or combine; wash, peel, core, and remove seeds if necessary; dice; and roast or steam (beets, squash, sweets only) until softened, then purée

Apple (any kind) or applesauce

Pear (any kind)

Banana

Beets (any kind), roasted or steamed

Butternut squash, roasted or steamed

Sweet potato, roasted or steamed

½ TO 1 TEASPOON TOTAL

Choose one

Apple cider vinegar

Fresh citrus juice

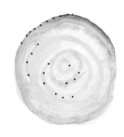
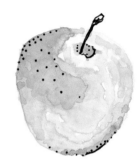

Flavor

Choose one or combine, or skip altogether

½ to 2 teaspoons extract (vanilla, almond, chocolate, peppermint, hazelnut)

½ to 2 teaspoons grated citrus zest

Seeds from ½ or 1 vanilla bean pod

½ to 2 teaspoons peeled, minced fresh ginger

1 to 3 teaspoons ground coffee or chicory root tea

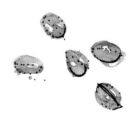

---

3 Fold together the wet and dry ingredients until mixed, then incorporate Fold-Ins (if using) until evenly distributed throughout. Use a spoon to place 1½-inch (4 cm) dollops of dough onto the lined baking sheet about 2 inches (5 cm) apart. Bake for 15 to 20 minutes, until browned and the tops and edges are cooked. Remove from the oven and cool on the baking sheet. The cookies will set more as they cool.

Fold-Ins

¼ TO ½ CUP TOTAL

Choose one or combine, or skip altogether

Coconut, shredded or flaked

Crystallized ginger, chopped

Dried fruit (cherries, dates, cranberries)

Nuts and/or seeds— raw or toasted

Dairy-free chocolate (dark or white chocolate bar; chopped or chips)

Hazelnut-Cranberry Cookies

Toasty hazelnuts and sweet-tart pops of cranberry—
a favorite to serve over the holidays. Fill them
with vanilla bean Nice Cream (page 279) for an extra special
ice-cream-sandwich-style treat!

MAKES 16 TO 18 COOKIES

½ cup (65 g) raw,
unsalted hazelnuts

¾ cup (150 g) coconut sugar

½ cup plus 2 tablespoons (70 g)
blanched almond flour

¼ cup (40 g) brown rice flour

¼ cup (30 g) sorghum flour

1 tablespoon arrowroot
starch/flour

1 teaspoon baking powder

½ teaspoon sea salt

¼ cup (60 g) applesauce

3 tablespoons warm water

2 tablespoons unrefined coconut
oil, gently warmed to liquid

1 teaspoon apple cider vinegar

1 teaspoon vanilla extract

½ cup (80 g) dried cranberries
(naturally sweetened)

1   Preheat the oven to 350°F (180°C) and line two large baking sheets with
    unbleached parchment paper or silicone baking mats. Place the hazelnuts
    on one baking sheet and roast for 7 to 10 minutes, until brown and smelling
    incredible. Remove from the oven and set aside.

2   In a large bowl, sift together the sugar, almond flour, rice flour, sorghum
    flour, arrowroot, baking powder, and salt.

3   In another large bowl, whisk together the applesauce, water, oil, vinegar,
    and vanilla extract until thoroughly combined.

4   Fold together the wet ingredients and flour mixture and incorporate the
    cranberries and hazelnuts until evenly distributed through the dough.

5   Use a spoon to place 1½-inch (4 cm) dollops of dough onto the lined baking
    sheets about 2 inches (5 cm) apart. Bake for 15 to 20 minutes, until browned
    and the tops and edges are cooked. Remove from the oven and cool on the
    baking sheets. The cookies will set more as they cool.

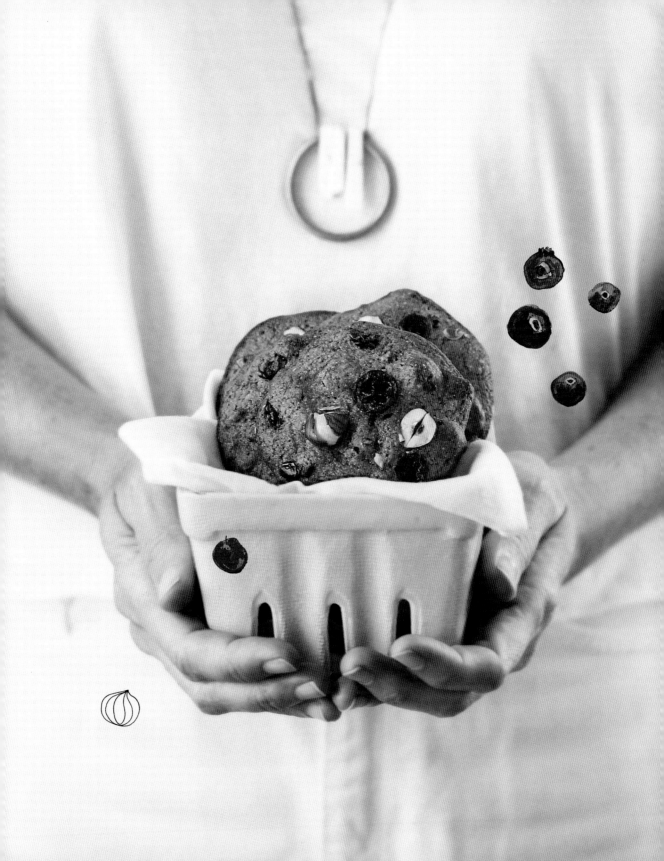

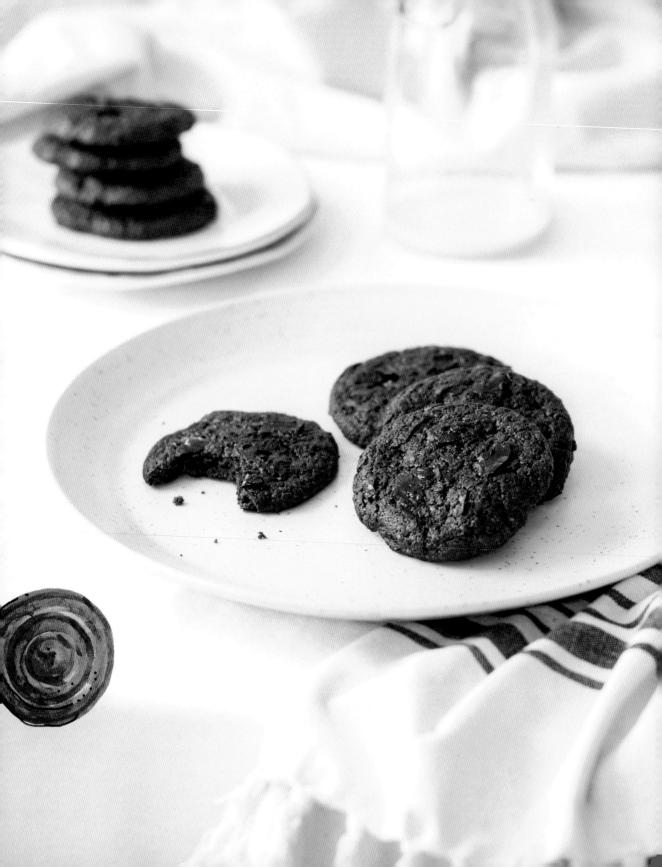

"Red Velvet" Peppermint Choco-Chip Cookies

A great one to try on all the "I don't like beets" people in your life. Not only do they provide beautiful "red velvet" color without chem-y dye, but they add a scrumptious level of sweetness to these cookies.

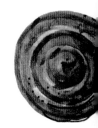

MAKES 16 TO 18 COOKIES

1 medium red beet, peeled and diced

3 tablespoons warm water, plus 1 to 2 tablespoons if needed

¾ cup (150 g) Sucanat

½ cup plus 2 tablespoons (70 g) blanched almond flour

½ cup (80 g) brown rice flour

2 tablespoons cocoa/cacao powder

1 tablespoon arrowroot starch/flour

1 teaspoon baking powder

½ teaspoon sea salt

2 tablespoons unrefined coconut oil, gently warmed to liquid

1 teaspoon peppermint extract

½ teaspoon vanilla extract

½ cup (85 g) chopped dark chocolate (one 3-ounce/85 g bar)

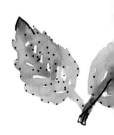

1   Preheat the oven to 350°F (180°C) and line two large baking sheets with unbleached parchment paper or silicone baking mats. Set aside, then start a double boiler and steam the diced beet until easily pierced with a fork.

2   Place the beet in the blender and purée, adding 1 to 2 tablespoons water if needed (just to get the blades going—you want applesauce consistency, not watery). Transfer ¼ cup (60 g) of the purée to a small bowl and save any leftover for Soup (page 175) or Muffins (page 63).

3   In a large bowl, sift together the Sucanat, almond flour, rice flour, cocoa powder, arrowroot, baking powder, and salt.

4   In another large bowl, whisk together 3 tablespoons warm water with the beet, oil, and peppermint and vanilla extracts until thoroughly combined.

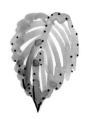

5   Fold together the wet ingredients and flour mixture, then incorporate the chocolate until evenly distributed. Use a spoon to place 1½-inch (4 cm) dollops of dough onto the lined baking sheets about 2 inches apart. Bake for 15 to 20 minutes, until browned and the tops and edges are cooked. Remove from the oven and cool on the baking sheets. The cookies will set more as they cool.

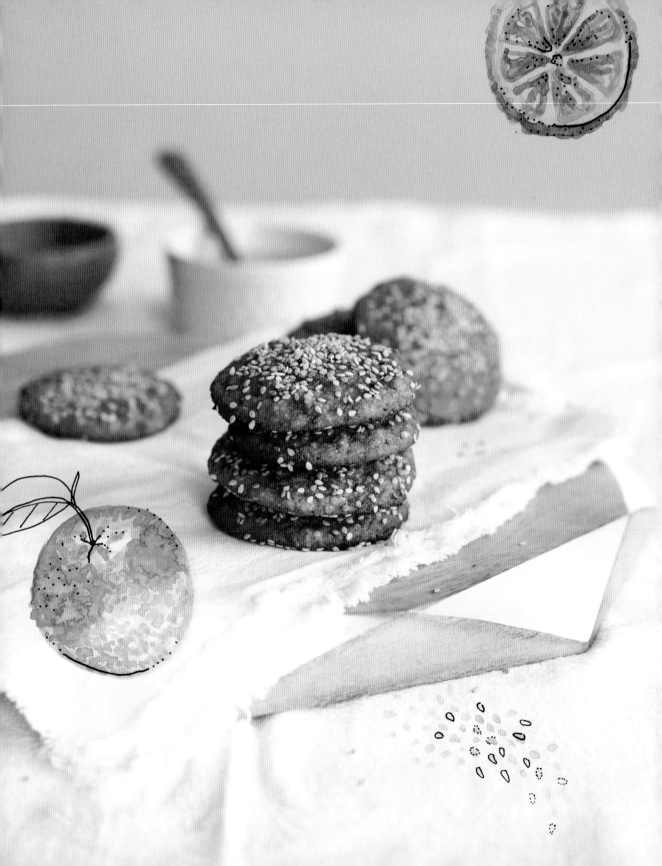

Sesame & Orange Cookies

A tasty combination of floral honey, toasted sesame, and brown-sugary sweetness from Sucanat makes this a simple cookie you'll love. Also delicious with 1 to 2 tablespoons of nutty tahini stirred in with the wet ingredients.

MAKES 16 TO 18 COOKIES

¼ cup (35 g) raw sesame seeds

¾ cup (150 g) Sucanat

½ cup plus 2 tablespoons (70 g) blanched almond flour

½ cup (60 g) millet flour

1 tablespoon arrowroot starch/flour

1 teaspoon baking powder

½ teaspoon sea salt

¼ cup (60 g) applesauce

3 tablespoons warm water

2 tablespoons unrefined coconut oil, gently warmed to liquid

1½ teaspoons grated orange zest

1 teaspoon fresh orange juice

1 teaspoon vanilla extract

1. Preheat the oven to 350°F (180°C) and line two large baking sheets with unbleached parchment paper or silicone baking mats. Set aside 1 tablespoon of the sesame seeds and scatter the remaining 3 tablespoons on a lined baking sheet to toast for 5 to 7 minutes, until lightly browned and smelling nutty. Set them aside, separate from the untoasted seeds.

2. In a large bowl, sift together the Sucanat, almond flour, millet flour, arrowroot, baking powder, and salt.

3. In another large bowl, whisk together the applesauce, water, oil, orange zest, orange juice, and vanilla extract until thoroughly combined.

4. Fold together the wet ingredients and flour mixture and incorporate the toasted sesame seeds. Use a spoon to place 1½-inch (4 cm) dollops of dough on the lined baking sheets about 2 inches (5 cm) apart. Sprinkle the tops generously with the untoasted sesame seeds. Bake for 15 to 20 minutes, until browned and the tops and edges are cooked. Remove from the oven and cool on the baking sheets. The cookies will set more as they cool.

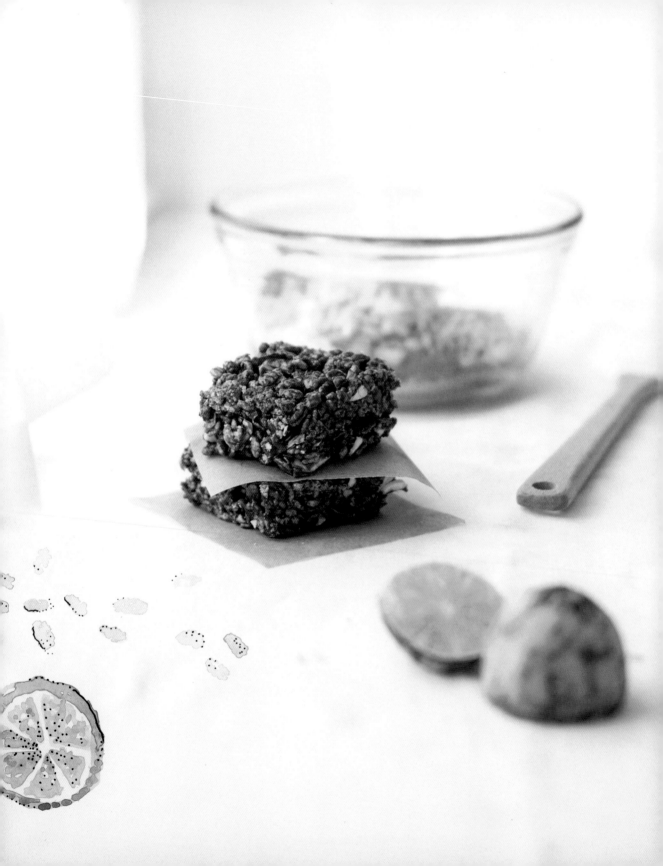

Nice Crispy Bars

Calling all sweet tooths: This is a sticky-sweet, gelatin-free twist on a classic childhood favorite we all know and love. Elevate them with crunchy additions like toasted coconut and unexpected flavors like tea. Shape them into hearts by hand, use cookie cutters to make circles, or roll them into bite-sized poppers like Amazeballs (page 121)—dip or drizzle with melted chocolate. Just make sure you use "crisp" cereals for your Crispies instead of "puffed" if you want that nostalgic crunch.

Nice Crispy Bar combo on this spread:
Cocoa, chocolate, cayenne, cinnamon, vanilla, lime zest & cashew.

Nice Crispy Bars

MAKES 12 TO 16 TREATS
COOK TIME: 10 TO 15 MINUTES

A few tips: If you use chocolate chips, know that they will melt from heat—yum! I use an 8-inch (20 cm) square baking dish or 8 x 4-inch (20 x 10 cm) loaf pan. You can grease it or line it with unbleached parchment before filling; once cooled, you can easily lift treats out and slice. And I highly recommend using a silicone spatula for stirring and ingredient transfer.

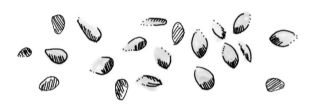

What you need no matter what:

¾ cup (180 ml) brown rice syrup

¼ teaspoon sea salt

1 In a large mixing bowl, stir together Crispies, Nuts & Seeds (if using), and Texture (if using) until thoroughly combined; set aside.

Crispies

3 CUPS (90 G) TOTAL
Choose one or combine

Crispy brown
rice cereal

Cocoa crispy brown
rice cereal

Sprouted crispy
brown rice cereal

Nuts & Seeds

½ TO 1 CUP TOTAL
Choose one or combine or skip altogether; all raw, unsalted

Chop medium to large nuts

Almonds	Macadamia nuts
Brazil nuts	Pecans
Cashews	Pepitas
Sunflower seeds	Pine nuts
Hazelnuts	Walnuts

Use only 1 to 2 tablespoons each of these in a mix

Chia seeds

Flaxseeds

Hemp seeds

Poppy seeds

Sesame seeds

Texture

Choose one to three or skip altogether

½ to 1 cup (40 to 80 g) shredded or flaked dried coconut

1 to 2 cups dried, dehydrated, or freeze-dried fruit (pome, berries, tropical)

½ cup (85 g) hulled buckwheat groats

¼ to ½ cup (25 to 50 g) brown rice flakes or quinoa flakes

¼ to ½ cup oats (old-fashioned rolled or steel cut)

¼ to ½ cup (10 to 15 g) popped/puffed grains (amaranth, brown rice, millet, quinoa)

½ to 1 cup (90 to 180 g) chopped chocolate or chocolate chips (dark or white)

¼ to ½ cup (15 to 30 g) crystallized ginger, chopped

---

2 Lightly grease a rectangular glass baking dish with Oil or line with unbleached parchment paper; set aside. In a large pot heated to medium, stir together the **brown rice syrup,** Second Sweet, Flavors, and the **salt** and bring to a vigorous boil—it has to reach this point for the treats to stick together. Reduce the heat and simmer and stir for 3 minutes so the sweetener thickens. Add the dry ingredients to the pot and stir together until evenly combined. Spoon into the dish, cool for 1 to 2 minutes, and, with greased hands, press into a firm layer. Chill in the fridge for 1 hour, slice, and enjoy. Store in the fridge for 2 to 3 weeks.

Oil

1 TEASPOON

Choose one

Unrefined coconut oil

Grapeseed oil

Sunflower seed oil

Second Sweet

¼ CUP TOTAL

Choose one

¼ cup (60 ml) raw, unpasteurized honey

¼ cup (60 ml) maple syrup

¼ cup (50 g) Sucanat

¼ cup (50 g) coconut sugar

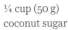

Flavor

Choose one or combine

2 to 4 tablespoons cacao nibs

¼ teaspoon ground cardamom

¼ teaspoon cayenne pepper

1 to 2 teaspoons ground cinnamon

¼ teaspoon ground cloves

¼ teaspoon ground nutmeg

1 to 2 teaspoons extract (almond, chocolate, hazelnut, vanilla)

1 to 2 tablespoons tea leaves, ground in coffee/spice grinder (chai, chicory root, Earl Grey, green, licorice root, rooibos, matcha, etc.)

1 to 6 teaspoons grated citrus zest

1 to 3 tablespoons cocoa/cacao powder

2 tablespoons ground coffee

1 to 2 tablespoons nut or seed butter

1 teaspoon orange blossom or rosewater

½ to 1 teaspoon ground ginger (or 1 to 2 teaspoons peeled, minced fresh ginger)

2 tablespoons jam

Coconut-y Hazelnut & Chai Crunch Bars

Chai tea, hazelnuts, toasty coconut, and pops of crystallized ginger make this a spicy, complex, and warming treat that feels special with every bite.

MAKES 12 TO 16 TREATS

Unrefined coconut oil for greasing (optional)

1 cup (85 g) dried, flaked coconut

½ cup (65 g) raw, unsalted hazelnuts

Pinch plus ¼ teaspoon sea salt

3 cups (90 g) crispy brown rice cereal

½ cup (80 g) crystallized ginger, chopped

¾ cup (180 ml) brown rice syrup

¼ cup (60 ml) maple syrup

2 teaspoons unsweetened chai tea leaves, ground in coffee/spice grinder

1 teaspoon vanilla extract

1. Lightly grease a rectangular glass baking dish with the oil, or line it with parchment paper.

2. Preheat the oven to 350°F (180°C). Line a baking sheet with unbleached parchment paper, spread the coconut in one layer, and toast for 3 to 5 minutes. Transfer three-fourths of the coconut to a large mixing bowl and set the rest aside. Spread the hazelnuts in one layer on the sheet. Sprinkle with a pinch of salt and pop in the oven for 7 minutes. Remove and cool, then slip off any loose hazelnut skins and discard. Chop and transfer to the large bowl. Add the cereal and ginger to the mixing bowl and toss.

3. In a large pot heated to medium, stir together the brown rice syrup, maple syrup, chai tea, vanilla extract, and remaining ¼ teaspoon salt and bring to a vigorous boil—it has to reach this point for the treats to stick together. Reduce the heat; simmer and stir for 3 minutes so the sweetener thickens. Turn off the heat and add the cereal mixture to the pot; use a silicone spatula to stir until thoroughly combined. Spoon into the baking dish. Cool for 1 to 2 minutes, then use greased hands to press into a firm layer. Sprinkle the remaining toasted coconut on top and press so they stick. Chill in the fridge for 1 hour, slice, and enjoy. Store in the fridge for weeks.

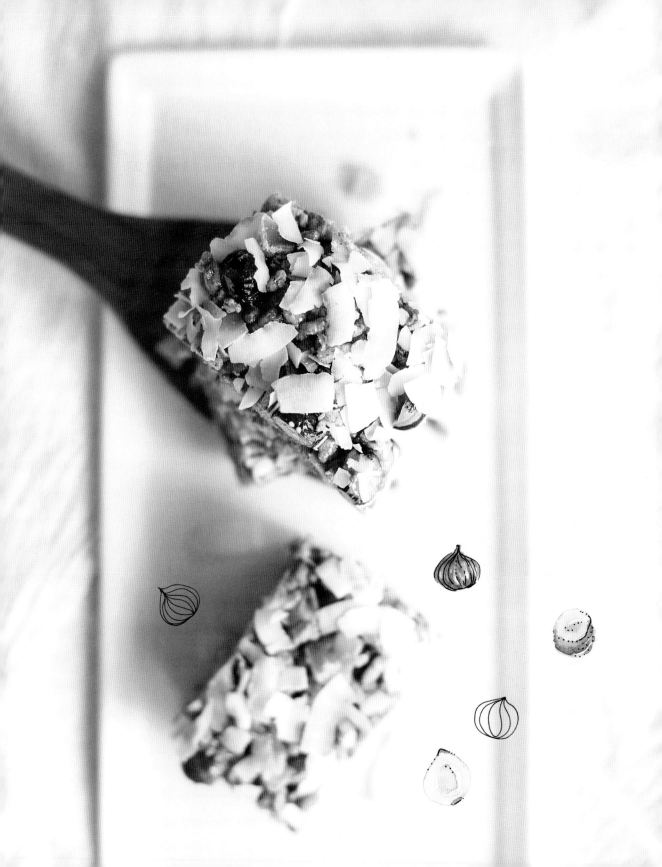

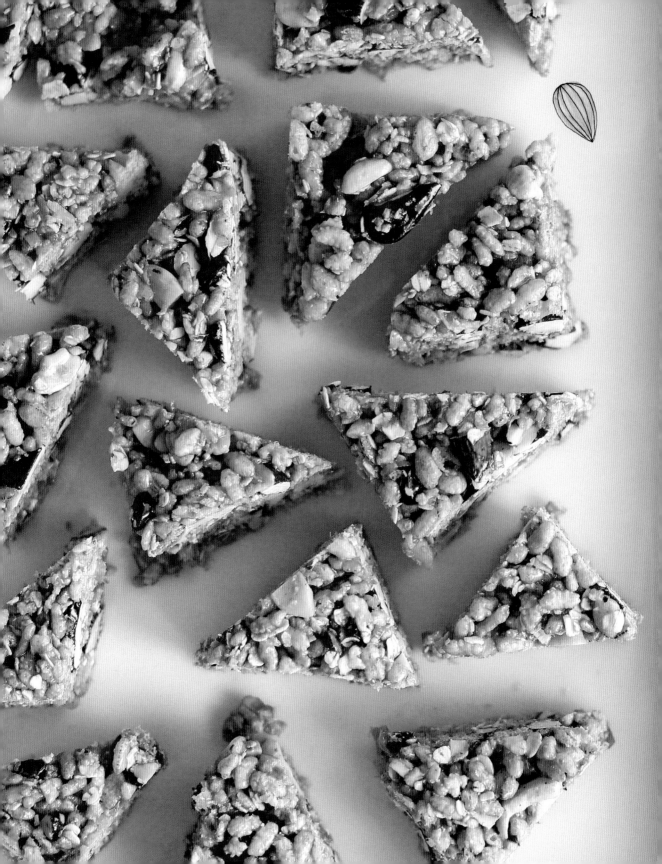

Orange Cream & Almond Crispy Bars

Inspired by the flavors of the childhood ice-cream-truck treat, this crispy dessert warms the heart and serves up some protein, too. Feel free to skip the orange blossom water if you like—it's just a fancy-pants addition if you have some in the kitchen.

MAKES 12 TO 16 TREATS

Unrefined coconut oil for greasing (optional)

¾ cup (110 g) raw, unsalted almonds

Pinch plus ¼ teaspoon sea salt

3 cups (90 g) crispy brown rice cereal

½ cup (70 g) raw, unsalted cashews, chopped

½ cup (40 g) rolled oats

¾ cup (180 ml) brown rice syrup

¼ cup (60 ml) raw, unpasteurized honey

2 tablespoons grated orange zest

1 tablespoon cashew butter

2 teaspoons vanilla extract

½ teaspoon orange blossom water (optional)

1. Lightly grease a rectangular baking dish with the oil, or line with unbleached parchment.

2. Preheat the oven to 350°F (180°C). Line a baking sheet with unbleached parchment paper, spread the almonds in one layer, sprinkle with a pinch of salt, and toast for 5 to 7 minutes; roughly chop and transfer to a large mixing bowl with the crispy brown rice cereal, cashews, and oats.

3. In a large pot heated to medium, stir together the brown rice syrup, honey, orange zest, cashew butter, vanilla extract, orange blossom water (if using), and remaining ¼ teaspoon salt and bring to a vigorous boil—it has to reach this point for the treats to stick together. Reduce the heat; simmer and stir for 3 minutes so the sweetener thickens. Turn off the heat and add the cereal mixture to the pot; use a silicone spatula to stir until thoroughly combined. Spoon into the baking dish. Cool for 1 to 2 minutes, then use greased hands to press into a firm layer. Chill in the fridge for 1 hour, slice, and enjoy. Store in the fridge for weeks.

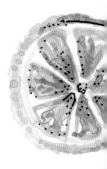

Neapolitan Nice Crispy Bars

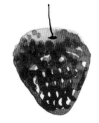

Let's divide the entire batch into thirds for flavored layers—
dish washing involved, but it's worth it!

MAKES 12 TO 16 TREATS

3 cups (90 g) crispy brown rice cereal

¾ cup (135 g) chocolate chips

1 cup (30 g) freeze-dried strawberries, chopped very fine

Unrefined coconut oil for greasing (optional)

¾ cup (180 ml) brown rice syrup

¼ cup (60 ml) raw, unpasteurized honey

1½ teaspoons vanilla extract

A few pinches sea salt

2 tablespoons strawberry jam

1 In each of two small bowls, place 1 cup of the crispy brown rice cereal. Add the chocolate chips to one bowl and the strawberries to the other.

2 Lightly grease an 8 x 4-inch (20 x 10 cm) glass loaf pan with the oil, or line it with parchment paper. In a large pot heated to medium, stir together ¼ cup (60 ml) of the brown rice syrup, 1 tablespoon plus 1 teaspoon of the honey, ½ teaspoon of the vanilla extract, and a pinch of the salt and bring to a vigorous boil—it has to reach this point for the treats to stick together. Reduce the heat; simmer and stir for 3 minutes so the sweetener thickens. Turn off the heat and, using a silicone spatula, stir in the chocolate-chip-cereal mixture. Transfer to the loaf pan and spread to fill the bottom. Cool for 2 minutes, then use greased hands to press into a firm layer.

3 Wash and dry the pot; stir together ¼ cup (60 ml) of the brown rice syrup, 1 tablespoon plus 1 teaspoon of the honey, ½ teaspoon of the vanilla extract, and a pinch of salt and bring to a boil. Reduce the heat; simmer and stir for 3 minutes. Turn off the heat and stir in the remaining 1 cup brown rice cereal (without the strawberries). Transfer to the loaf pan, and spread to cover the chocolate layer. Cool for 2 minutes, then press into a firm layer.

4 Last time: Wash and dry the pot; stir together the remaining brown rice syrup, honey, vanilla extract, pinch of salt, and the strawberry jam and bring to a boil. Reduce the heat; simmer and stir for 3 minutes. Turn off the heat and stir in the strawberry-cereal mixture. Transfer to the loaf pan, cover the vanilla layer, and cool for 2 minutes; press into a firm layer. Chill for 1 hour, slice, and enjoy. Store in the fridge for weeks.

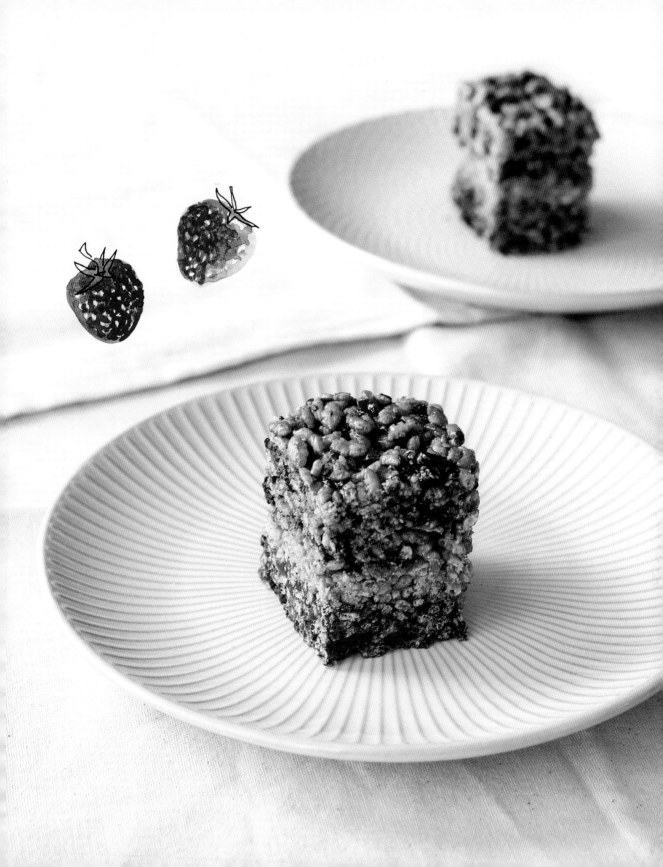

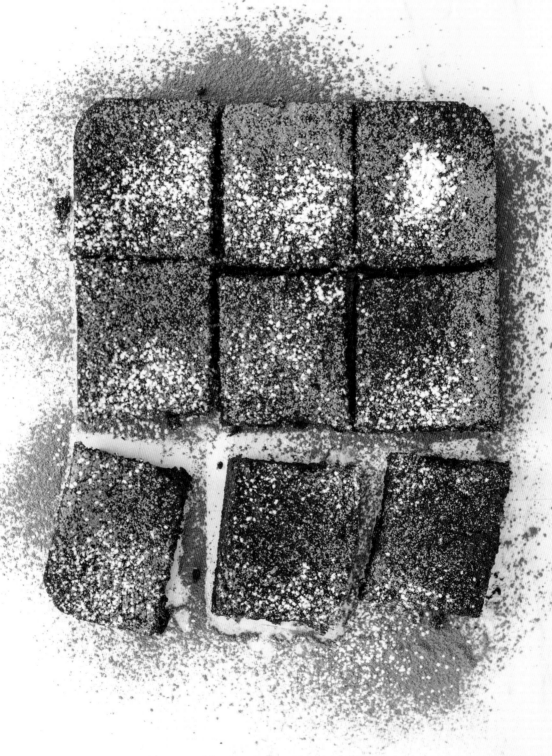

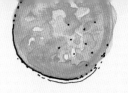

Sneaky Brownies

These brownies are rich, decadent cake-like squares
of goodness with nutrient-dense ingredients
such as beets, carrots, and summer squash snuck into
the mix (so stealthy, they'll never know!).
Not only will you be surprised at how delicious veggies
in desserts can be, but the kiddos and veg skeptics
in your life will be, too.

Sneaky Brownie combo on this spread:
Chopped chocolate bar, Ceylon cinnamon & butternut squash.

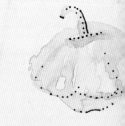

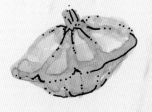

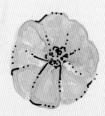

Sneaky Brownies

MAKES 12+
COOK TIME: 15 TO 35 MINUTES

You can use raw cacao powder or dairy-free cocoa powder in equal amounts for this template. I call for blanched almond flour in all variations because it adds protein and a nice cakey crumb.

Prefer a nut-free brownie? Substitute almond flour with equal amounts of Grain Flour. I also use our friend psyllium husk here because it binds so well. You'll need an 8- or 9-inch (20 or 23 cm) square baking dish. For more flavor, pretoast nuts and seeds for 7 minutes or coconut for 3 minutes before folding into the batter.

What you need no matter what:

½ cup (120 ml) unrefined coconut oil, gently warmed to liquid, plus more for greasing

¾ cup (85 g) blanched almond flour

½ cup (45 g) cocoa/cacao powder

1 teaspoon baking powder

1 teaspoon baking soda

¾ teaspoon ground psyllium husk

½ teaspoon sea salt

1 to 2 tablespoons water

½ cup (120 ml) warm water or dairy-free milk

1 Preheat the oven to 350°F (180°C); grease a baking dish with the **oil.** In a large bowl, stir together Sweet, Grain Flour, the **almond flour, cocoa/cacao powder, baking powder, baking soda, psyllium, salt,** and Flavor (if using).

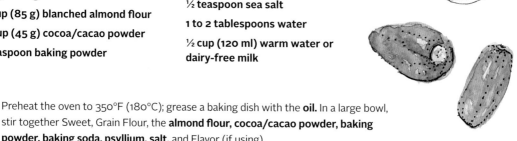

Sweet ----- *and* ----> Grain Flour

¾ CUP (150 G) TOTAL
Choose one or combine

Sucanat

Rapadura

Coconut sugar

¾ CUP TOTAL
Choose at least two and mix

Oat flour

Sorghum flour

Gluten-free all-purpose flour

Brown rice flour

Flavor

Choose one or combine, or skip altogether

1 to 2 teaspoons extract (vanilla, almond, cocoa, hazelnut)

¼ cup (20 g) fine-ground coffee

Seeds from 1 vanilla bean pod

¼ to 1 teaspoon grated citrus zest

½ to 1 teaspoon ground cinnamon

¼ cup (35 g) roasted ground chicory root

Pinch to ¼ teaspoon ground cardamom

Pinch to ¼ teaspoon cayenne pepper

1 to 2 teaspoons chai tea leaves, ground in coffee/spice grinder

2 To make a purée, put Fruit & Veg in a blender, add the **water,** and blend until smooth. Transfer to another bowl and whisk together with ½ **cup (120 ml) oil** and the **water or dairy-free milk** until smooth. Pour into the large bowl of dry ingredients and fold together until thoroughly incorporated.

Fruit & Veg

1½ CUPS TOTAL
Choose one or combine

Apple (any kind), cored and diced, or applesauce

Banana

Beet (any kind), roasted or steamed

Winter squash, roasted or steamed

Pumpkin, roasted or steamed

Sweet potato, roasted or steamed

Summer squash

Carrots, roasted or steamed

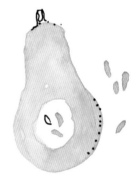

3 Incorporate dry Fold-Ins (if using) and spread in the baking dish. If using wet Fold-Ins, spread the batter in the baking dish and then swirl in the wet Fold-Ins. Bake for 25 to 35 minutes, until the edges and center are dry. Cool entirely in the dish, slice, and enjoy. Store in the fridge for a few weeks, or freeze for a few months.

Fold-Ins

¼ TO ½ CUP TOTAL
Choose one or combine, or skip altogether

*Dry ingredients **AND/OR*** ---------------→ *Wet ingredients*

¾ to 1 cup (60 to 80 g) shredded or flaked dried coconut

¾ to 1 cup (135 to 180 g) chocolate chips or chopped chocolate (white or dark)

1 to 2 tablespoons chia seeds

¾ cup (105 g) nuts and/or seeds, toasted

¾ cup (120 g) dried fruit (dates, cherries)

¼ to ½ cup (80 to 160 g) fruit purée or Compote (page 90)

¼ to ½ cup (80 to 160 g) jam or jelly (berries, apricot, cherries)

¼ to ½ cup (60 to 120 g) Probiotic Cream Cheese (page 128)

¼ to ½ cup (60 to 120 ml) Butterscotch (page 33)

3 tablespoons maple syrup

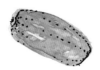

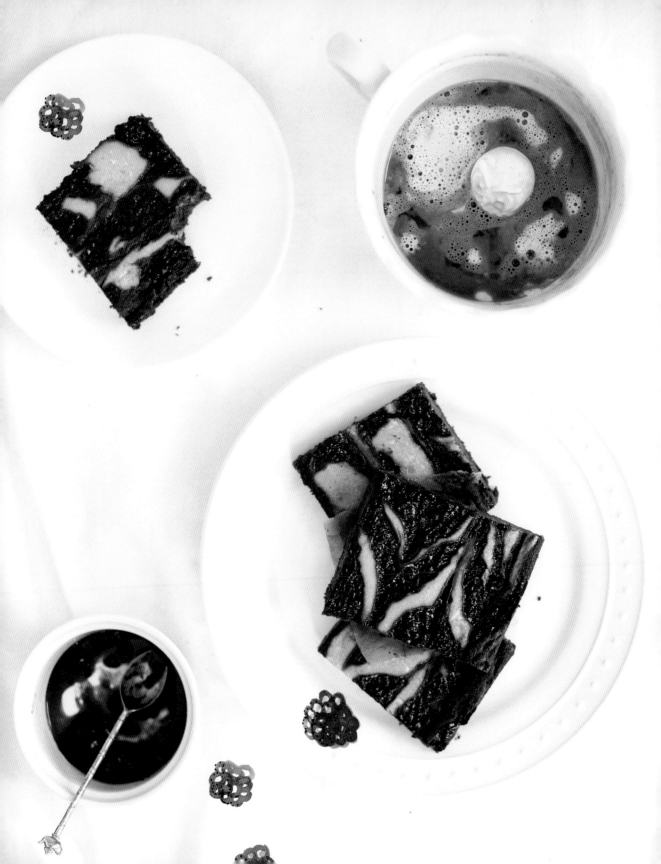

Raspberry & Cream Cheese Swirl Brownies

Dark chocolate, sweet, juicy raspberries, and sour homemade Cream Cheese (page 128)—yep, cream cheese—a truly scrumptious combo.

MAKES 12+

½ cup (120 g) unsweetened Probiotic Cream Cheese (page 128) or any store-bought dairy-free cream cheese you like

1 cup (200 g) plus 1 tablespoon coconut sugar

1 to 3 tablespoons water

½ cup (120 ml) unrefined coconut oil, gently warmed to liquid, plus more for greasing

¾ cup (85 g) blanched almond flour

¾ cup (90 g) sorghum flour

½ cup (40 g) cocoa/cacao powder

1 teaspoon baking powder

1 teaspoon baking soda

¾ teaspoon ground psyllium husk

½ teaspoon sea salt

1½ cups (360 g) applesauce

½ cup (120 ml) warm water

2 teaspoons vanilla extract

1 cup (320 g) raspberry Compote (page 90) or raspberry jam

1. Whisk together the Probiotic Cream Cheese, 1 tablespoon of the sugar, and enough of the water to make the cheese a thick but swirlable, pourable consistency—think creamy, melted ice cream.

2. Preheat the oven to 350°F (180°C). Grease an 8- or 9-inch (20 or 23 cm) square baking dish with a small amount of oil and set aside. In a large bowl, stir together the remaining 1 cup (200 g) sugar, the almond flour, sorghum flour, cocoa powder, baking powder, baking soda, psyllium, and salt.

3. Whisk together the applesauce, oil, warm water, and vanilla extract. Pour into the dry ingredients and fold together until thoroughly incorporated.

4. Spread the batter in the baking dish and spoon or pour the cream cheese in lines across the batter. Do the same with the raspberry compote in between the cream cheese lines. Run a knife perpendicular to the lines to swirl together. Bake for 30 to 35 minutes, until the edges and center are dry. Cool entirely in the dish, slice, and enjoy. Store in the fridge for a few weeks, or freeze for a few months.

Mocha, Almond & Chocolate Chunk Brownies

Roasted chicory root tea is a nice caffeine-free substitute
for coffee in these brownies if you want to change it up.
Be sure to source a gluten-free, vegan chocolate bar if you have
sensitivities. I highly recommend serving warm with
vanilla Nice Cream (page 280) and/or Butterscotch (page 33).

MAKES 12+

¾ cup (110 g) raw, unsalted almonds

Pinch plus ½ teaspoon salt

½ cup (120 ml) unrefined coconut oil, gently warmed to liquid, plus more for greasing

1¼ cup (200 g) brown rice flour

1 cup (200 g) Sucanat

¾ cup (85 g) blanched almond flour

½ cup (25 g) cocoa/cacao powder

1 teaspoon baking powder

1 teaspoon baking soda

¾ teaspoon ground psyllium husk

1½ cups (195 g) diced carrots, steamed and puréed

½ cup (120 ml) warm water

3 tablespoons maple syrup

2 teaspoons vanilla extract

1 cup (170 g) chopped dark chocolate (one to two 3-ounce/85 g bars)

¼ cup (20 g) fine-ground coffee

1. Preheat the oven to 350°F (180°C) and line a baking sheet with unbleached parchment paper. Scatter the almonds in one layer on the sheet and sprinkle with a pinch of salt. Roast for 7 minutes, remove, cool, chop, and set aside.

2. Grease an 8- or 9-inch (20 to 23 cm) square baking dish with oil. In a large bowl, stir together the rice flour, Sucanat, almond flour, cocoa powder, baking powder, baking soda, psyllium, and the remaining ½ teaspoon salt.

3. In another bowl, whisk together the carrot purée, oil, water, maple syrup, and vanilla extract. Pour into the dry ingredients and mix together until thoroughly incorporated, then fold in the chocolate, coffee, and almonds. Spread in the baking dish and bake for 25 to 35 minutes, until the edges and center are dry. Cool entirely in the dish, slice, and enjoy. Store in the fridge for a few weeks, or freeze for a few months.

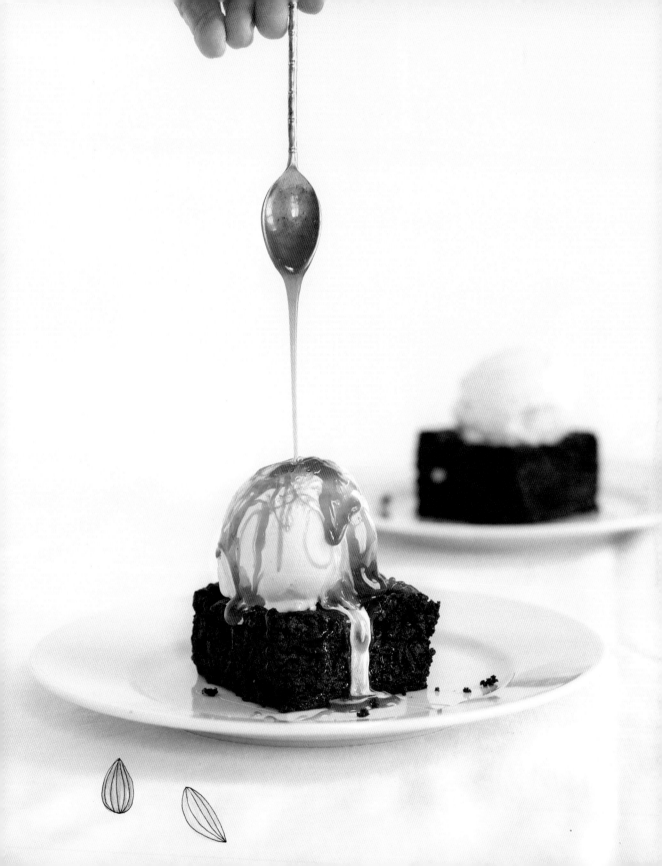

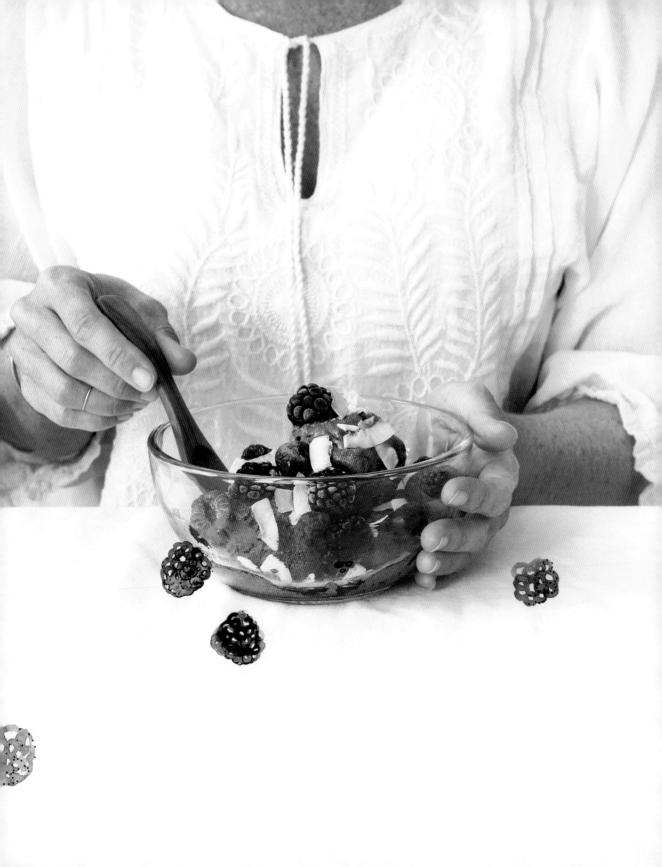

Nice Cream

This is my go-to template for creamy, unforgettable dairy-free ice cream. You can make a variety of decadent flavors with this base, and I do recommend an ice cream maker for the best aeration, but it's not required. Just freeze what you have—it'll still be tasty.

Play with out-of-the-box preparations like roasting or grilling fruit before folding into the base. And note that honey lends a nice, light color to ice cream, while dark sweeteners give it a caramel hue. A sweetener like molasses has bold flavor—let it be the hero.

Put a scoop of Nice Cream on a Sneaky Brownie (page 271), drizzle with Butterscotch (page 33) and/or Compote (page 90), and top it all with toasted nuts and/or coconut—sundae time!

Nice Cream combo on this spread: Raspberry, honey & fresh beet juice.

Nice Cream

4+ SERVINGS
PREP TIME: 15 TO 35 MINUTES

Canned, full-fat coconut milk is the way to go—even the most die-hard "I don't like coconut" peeps ask for "just a little more, please."

Until you're comfy combining flavors, keep it simple—I've got suggestions to get you started with either a vanilla (V) or chocolate (C) base. If you don't have arrowroot, you can skip it, but it helps minimize ice crystals while maximizing effortless scoopability.

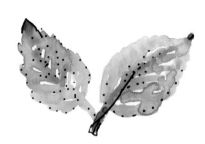

What you need no matter what:

3 cups (720 ml) canned full-fat coconut milk

1 tablespoon arrowroot starch/flour

1 tablespoon unrefined coconut oil (optional, but adds nice texture to the base)

¼ teaspoon sea salt

1 In a large pot heated to medium-high, whisk together the **coconut milk,** Sweet to taste, the **arrowroot, oil** (if using), and **salt** until velvety smooth and starting to simmer. Remove from the heat and transfer to a blender with one Base; blend for 2 to 3 minutes, until velvety smooth. If you don't have an ice cream maker, blend for a total of 5 minutes to aerate.

Sweet ----- *and* ----→ Base

¼ TO ½ CUP TOTAL
Choose one or combine

Sucanat

Rapadura

Coconut sugar

Maple syrup

Raw, unpasteurized honey

Blackstrap molasses

Choose one

Vanilla base (V):

1 to 3 teaspoons vanilla extract

AND/OR

Seeds from 1 vanilla bean pod

Chocolate base (C):

¼ cup (20 g) cocoa/cacao powder

AND (if you like)

Seeds from 1 vanilla bean pod

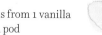

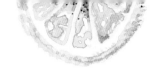

2 Blend in Flavor (if using), but stop after a few seconds to maintain flecks of color.

Flavor

UP TO ¼ CUP TOTAL

Choose one or two below, or skip altogether

1 to 3 teaspoons extract (almond, hazelnut, mint) **V**

1 to 3 teaspoons extract (vanilla, almond, cocoa, hazelnut, mint) **C**

¼ teaspoon orange blossom or rosewater **V**

¼ to 1 cup (60 to 240 g) Probiotic Cream Cheese (page 128) **V C**

1 teaspoon to 3 tablespoons grated lemon or lime zest **V**

1 teaspoon to 3 tablespoons grated orange zest **V C**

½ to 1 teaspoon fresh-cracked pepper (pink, white, black or Sichuan peppercorn) **V C**

½ to 1 teaspoon ground cardamom **V C**

¼ cup (60 ml) port, red wine, white wine, Champagne, Chambord, Cointreau, bourbon **V C**

¼ to 3 teaspoons ground cinnamon **V C**

¼ teaspoon chipotle powder **C**

¼ teaspoon cayenne pepper **C**

1 to 2 tablespoons tea leaves, ground in a coffee/spice grinder (chai, chicory root, Earl Grey, licorice root, rooibos, matcha) **V C**

2 tablespoons ground coffee **V C**

2 tablespoons pumpkin pie spice **V C**

1 teaspoon to 2 tablespoons peeled, minced fresh ginger **V C**

¼ teaspoon ground nutmeg **V C**

---

3 Using an ice cream maker? Chill the blended mixture for 3 hours in the fridge, then process in the machine until firm but stirrable. No ice cream maker? Freeze the mixture until firm but stirrable. Using a spoon, evenly distribute Fold-Ins (if using), maintaining swirls and chunks. Freeze for 2 to 3 hours until firm—thaw to scoop.

Fold-Ins

UP TO 2 CUPS TOTAL

Choose one or combine, or skip altogether

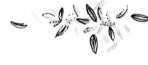

½ to 1 cup dried fruit (raisins, dates, cherries, cranberries) **V C**

½ to 1½ cups fresh fruit, mashed or chopped **V C**

¼ to 1 cup (35 to 135 g) sweet corn kernels (non-GMO) **V**

1 to 2 teaspoons fennel seed, toasted **V C**

¼ to ½ cup (20 to 40 g) cocoa/cacao powder **V C**

¼ to 1 cup (65 to 260 g) unsalted nut or seed butter **V C**

½ to 1 cup (70 to 140 g) chopped nuts & seeds, toasted **V C**

½ to 1 cup (40 to 80 g) flaked or shredded dried coconut **V C**

2 tablespoons to ¼ cup (60 ml) balsamic vinegar or reduction **V**

1 to 2 cups (85 to 170 g) Pie Crust Crumbles (page 286) or a sweet cracker from page 112, crumbled **V C**

¼ to 1 cup (60 to 240 ml) Butterscotch (page 33) **V C**

½ to 1 cup (90 to 180 g) chopped chocolate or chocolate chips (dark or white) **V C**

¼ to ½ cup (40 to 80 g) crystallized ginger, chopped **V C**

½ to 1½ cups (160 to 480 g) jam, Compote, or Fruit Butter (page 90) **V C**

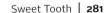

Blueberry Balsamic Nice Cream

If you haven't tried balsamic reduction on your ice cream yet—
let me tell you, the time is now. There's something
surprisingly addicting about that sweet acidity paired with a
creamy coconut base and juicy blueberries. This is simple,
next-level deliciousness.

SERVES 4+

3 cups (720 ml) canned
full-fat coconut milk

1½ cups (215 g) fresh blueberries

½ cup (100 g) coconut sugar

1 tablespoon arrowroot
starch/flour

1 tablespoon unrefined
coconut oil

1 teaspoon vanilla extract

½ teaspoon fresh thyme leaves
(optional)

¼ teaspoon sea salt

1 cup (240 ml) balsamic vinegar

1 Blend together the coconut milk and blueberries (or only a half or third
of the berries and fold in the rest after processing in the ice cream maker
for texture), then transfer to a large pot and heat to medium-high.

2 Whisk in the sugar, arrowroot, oil, vanilla extract, thyme (if using), and
salt until velvety smooth and starting to simmer. Remove from the heat
and chill for 2 to 3 hours in the fridge until thoroughly cool.

3 Let's make a balsamic reduction. Pour the balsamic vinegar into a pot and
bring to a boil over medium-high heat. Reduce the heat to medium-low
and simmer softly until the sauce reduces by 75 percent. Remove from the
heat and set aside—the reduction will thicken as it cools. Make sure it's
room temp or cooler when you ultimately swirl it into your ice cream.

4 Process the chilled milk mixture in an ice cream maker until firm but
stirrable. Transfer to a freezable container and fold in the balsamic
reduction until evenly distributed but not thoroughly incorporated—
you want swirls. Freeze for 1 to 3 hours, until firm. Thaw to scoopable
consistency and serve.

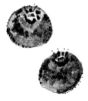

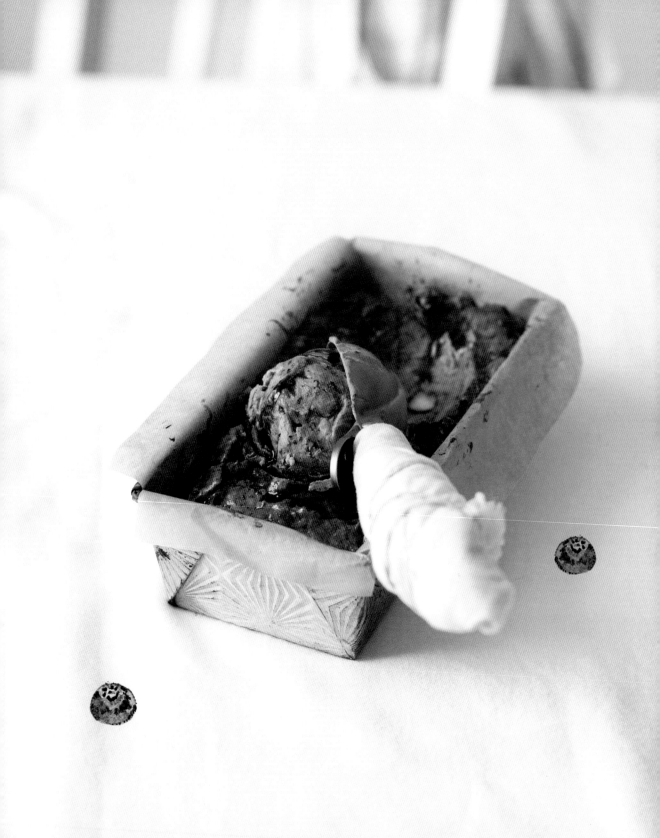

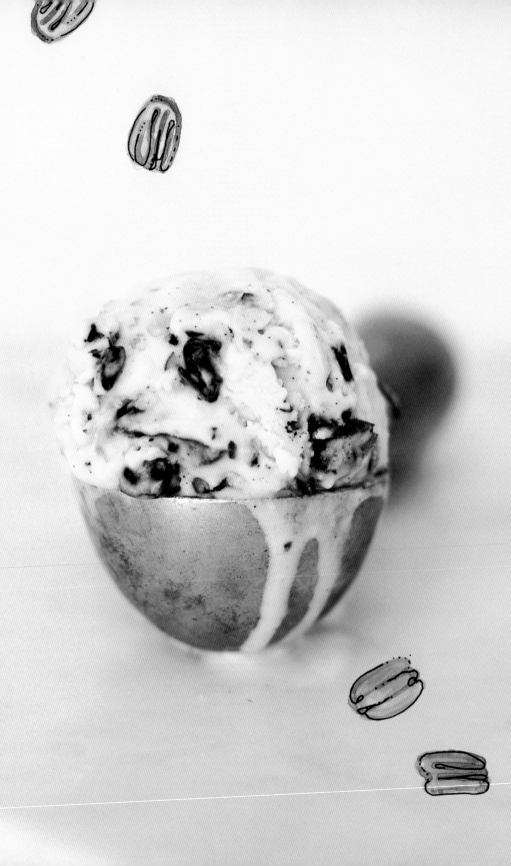

Bourbon Salted Chocolate-Pecan Cluster Nice Cream

This one is for my grandparents, who loved their bourbon, and their sweets. If you don't love a boozy kiss in a dessert, simply leave out the bourbon.

SERVES 4+

½ cup (50 g) raw pecan halves

1 tablespoon plus ½ cup (120 ml) maple syrup

½ teaspoon sea salt

¼ teaspoon ground cinnamon

Two pinches cayenne pepper

Two pinches ground cardamom (optional)

1 vanilla bean pod

3 cups (720 ml) canned full-fat coconut milk

1 tablespoon unrefined coconut oil

2 tablespoons bourbon

1 tablespoon arrowroot starch/flour

One 3-ounce (85 g) dark chocolate bar

1   Preheat the oven to 350°F (180°C) and line a baking sheet with unbleached parchment paper. In a small bowl, stir together the pecans, 1 tablespoon of the maple syrup, ¼ teaspoon of the salt, cinnamon, cayenne, and cardamom until the pecans are coated. Scatter on the baking sheet and roast for 7 to 10 minutes, until browned. Remove from the baking sheet and cool in the fridge.

2   Press the vanilla bean pod so it lies flat on a cutting board. Carefully slice down its entire length with a sharp knife and open. Use the back of your knife to scrape out the caviar-like seeds and toss into a large pot. Heat the pot to medium-high and whisk together the coconut milk, the remaining ½ cup (120 ml) maple syrup, oil, bourbon, arrowroot, and ¼ teaspoon salt until velvety smooth and starting to simmer. Remove from the heat and chill for 2 to 3 hours in the fridge, until thoroughly cool.

3   Melt the chocolate bar over a double boiler and toss the pecans in the chocolate until coated. Cool in the fridge; chop into bite-sized pieces.

4   Process the chilled milk mixture in an ice cream maker until firm but stirrable. Transfer to a freezable container and fold in the pecan clusters until evenly distributed but maintain swirls and chunks. Freeze for 1 to 3 hours, until firm. Thaw to scoopable consistency and serve.

Loaded Cherry Pie Nice Cream

If cherries aren't in season, try any other pie-worthy fruit.
Cardamom and rosewater add floral notes, but you can skip them.
If you do, try folding in a chopped chocolate bar instead.

SERVES 4+

Pie Crust Crumbles
(a sweet riff on the Cracker
template on page 112)

½ cup (55 g) blanched
almond flour

½ cup (80 g) brown rice flour

2 tablespoons Sucanat

¼ teaspoon baking powder

¼ teaspoon sea salt

1 tablespoon chilled unrefined
coconut oil

1 teaspoon vanilla extract

2 tablespoons cold water,
plus more if needed

—

3 cups (720 ml) canned
full-fat coconut milk

½ cup (120 ml) raw,
unpasteurized honey

1 tablespoon arrowroot
starch/flour

1 tablespoon unrefined
coconut oil

2 teaspoons vanilla extract

1 teaspoon fresh lemon juice

¼ teaspoon rosewater (optional)

¼ teaspoon sea salt

Pinch ground cardamom
(optional)

1½ cups (480 g) cherry Compote
(page 90)

1. For pie crust crumbles: Preheat the oven to 375°F (190°C). In a bowl using a fork, or in a food processor, mix together the almond flour, rice flour, Sucanat, baking powder, and salt. Cut in the chilled coconut oil and vanilla extract until crumbly. Cut in 1 tablespoon of the cold water. Form a ball of dough and use a rolling pin to flatten to ⅛ to ¼ inch (3 to 6 mm) between two sheets of parchment paper. Slide the dough and the bottom sheet of parchment onto a baking sheet and bake for 10 to 15 minutes, until the edges brown. Remove from the oven, cool, and break apart into bite-sized pieces.

2. For nice cream: In a pot heated to medium-high, whisk together the coconut milk, honey, arrowroot, coconut oil, vanilla extract, lemon juice, rosewater (if using), salt, and cardamom until smooth and starting to simmer. Remove from the heat and chill for 2 to 3 hours in the fridge, until thoroughly cool.

3. Process in an ice cream maker until firm but stirrable. Transfer to a freezable container and fold in the compote and pie crust crumbles until evenly distributed but not thoroughly incorporated—you want swirls and chunks. Freeze for 1 to 3 hours, until firm. Thaw to scoopable consistency and serve.

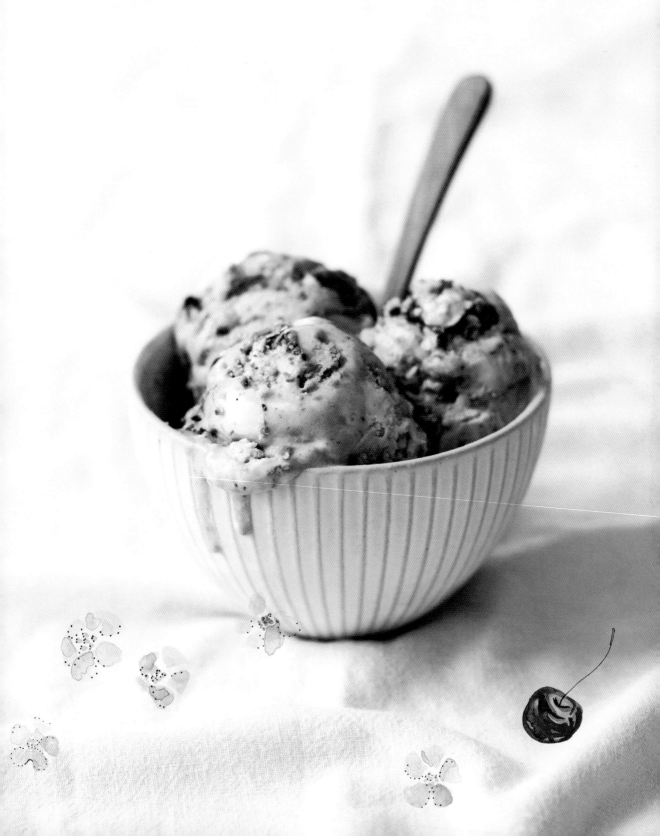

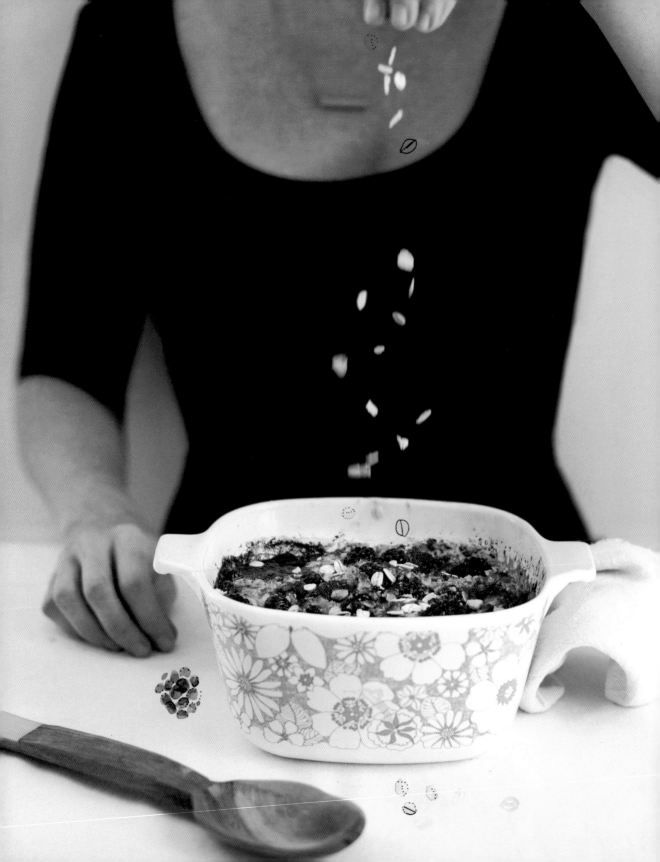

Crisps & Crumbles

Call it a "crisp" (contains oats) or a "crumble" (no oats) because there really isn't a popular consensus about the difference. It's simply all of the edible-hug-like flavor of pie, but easier to prepare. Bake up this fruity, crunchy goodness in a casserole dish or cast-iron skillet, or use ramekins for single-serving treats.

Keep it classic with combinations like mixed berries, or pome fruit and cinnamon. Add some fun with dollops of homemade Probiotic Cream Cheese (page 128), or go far on the creativity scale with some sweet root veggies and spice, or mixed berries with red wine or balsamic vinegar. Use more sugar and less lemon juice when cooking with tart fruits, like rhubarb and blackberries, and less sugar but more lemon juice for sweet fruits, like peaches and plums.

Just be sure to serve it warm, probably with homemade Nice Cream (page 279)—now that's a wise choice.

Crisp combo on this spread: Mixed berry & almond-oat topping.

Crisps & Crumbles

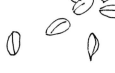

6+ SERVINGS
COOK TIME: 15 TO 40 MINUTES

Let your taste buds decide sweetness levels for the topping and fruit mixture—start with less and add more to taste. Keep in mind: Sweetness will amplify 15 to 20 percent as fruits cook down.

If they're new to you, quinoa flakes and brown rice flakes look just like rolled oats. They're sometimes sold in the cereal aisle.

What you need no matter what:

⅓ cup (80 ml) unrefined coconut oil, plus more for greasing (solid or liquid)

¾ teaspoon sea salt

2 teaspoons arrowroot flour/starch

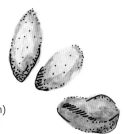

1 Preheat the oven to 375°F (190°C) and lightly grease a 10- to 12-inch (25 to 30 cm) cast-iron skillet or baking dish, or six to eight 4-inch (10 cm) ramekins with **oil** and set aside. In a medium bowl, use a fork to combine Texture, Flour, Topping Sweet, ⅓ **cup (80 ml) oil**, and ¼ **teaspoon salt** until crumbly; set aside this crumble mixture.

Texture --- *and* ---> Flour ------ *and* ----> Topping Sweet

1 CUP TOTAL
Choose one or combine

Rolled oats

Quinoa flakes

Raw, unsalted nuts, finely chopped

Brown rice flakes

Dried coconut (shredded or flakes)

¾ CUP TOTAL
Choose one or combine

Blanched almond flour

Brown rice flour

Oat flour

Gluten-free all-purpose flour

¼ CUP (50 G) TOTAL
Choose one or combine

Sucanat

Rapadura

Coconut sugar

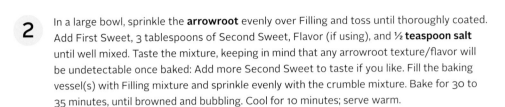

2   In a large bowl, sprinkle the **arrowroot** evenly over Filling and toss until thoroughly coated. Add First Sweet, 3 tablespoons of Second Sweet, Flavor (if using), and ½ **teaspoon salt** until well mixed. Taste the mixture, keeping in mind that any arrowroot texture/flavor will be undetectable once baked: Add more Second Sweet to taste if you like. Fill the baking vessel(s) with Filling mixture and sprinkle evenly with the crumble mixture. Bake for 30 to 35 minutes, until browned and bubbling. Cool for 10 minutes; serve warm.

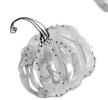

Filling

5 TO 6 CUPS TOTAL

Choose one or combine

Pome fruit, chopped or sliced (apple, pear, quince)

Berries (blackberry, blueberry, raspberry, strawberry)

Stone fruit, chopped or sliced (cherries, peaches, nectarines, plums)

Sweet potato, diced, steamed/roasted

Pumpkin, diced, steamed/roasted

First Sweet ------- *and* -------→ Second Sweet

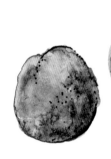
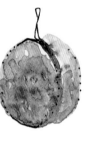

2 TABLESPOONS TOTAL

Choose one

Sucanat

Rapadura

Coconut sugar

3 TABLESPOONS TO ½ CUP TOTAL

Choose one or combine

Compote or Fruit Butter (page 90)

Jam or jelly

Blackstrap molasses

Brown rice syrup

Raw, unpasteurized honey

Maple syrup

Sucanat

Rapadura

Coconut sugar

Flavor

Optional

¼ teaspoon ground allspice

¼ teaspoon ground cardamom

1 to 2 teaspoons ground cinnamon

¼ teaspoon ground cloves

¼ to ½ cup (35 to 75 g) dried fruit (dates, raisins, cranberries)

¼ to ½ cup (25 to 50 g) fresh cranberries

¼ teaspoon fresh ground nutmeg

1 teaspoon extract (almond, hazelnut, vanilla)

1 to 2 teaspoons grated citrus zest

1 to 3 teaspoons fresh citrus juice

1 to 2 teaspoons apple cider vinegar

¼ teaspoon orange blossom water or rosewater

1 to 2 tablespoons booze (fruit brandy, dry red wine, bourbon, Chambord, Cointreau)

1 to 2 teaspoons balsamic vinegar

½ to 1½ teaspoons ground ginger (or 1 to 3 teaspoons peeled, minced fresh ginger)

¼ cup (60 g) Probiotic Cream Cheese (page 129)

1 to 2 teaspoons fresh thyme

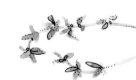

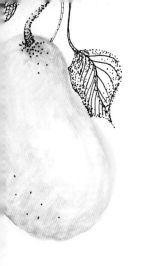

Apricot & Pear Crisp

In this recipe, we add flavor and sweetness by tossing fruit with apricot jam, and also adding some dried fruit for moments of chewy texture. This recipe is also nice with added dollops of Probiotic Cream Cheese before baking (page 128), but either way, serve warm with coconut cream, Nice Cream (page 279), and/or a drizzle of Butterscotch (page 33).

SERVES 6+

⅓ cup (80 ml) unrefined coconut oil, plus more for greasing (solid or liquid)

½ cup (75 g) raw, unsalted almonds, chopped finely

¼ cup (40 g) brown rice flour

¼ cup (20 g) flaked dried coconut

¼ cup (25 g) rolled oats

¼ cup (30 g) sorghum flour

¼ cup (60 g) plus 2 tablespoons Sucanat

¾ teaspoon sea salt

2 teaspoons arrowroot flour/starch

3 pears (Bosc, Bartlett or Anjou), peeled or skin on (chef's choice), sliced or diced (about 6 cups/480 g)

½ cup (160 g) apricot jam

½ cup (85 g) dried apricots, chopped

2 teaspoons fresh lemon juice

1 teaspoon almond extract

1 teaspoon vanilla extract

1. Preheat the oven to 375°F (190°C) and lightly grease a 10- to 12-inch (25 to 30 cm) round or square baking dish with coconut oil and set aside. In a medium bowl, use a fork to combine the oil, almonds, rice flour, coconut, oats, sorghum flour, ¼ cup (60 g) of the Sucanat, and ¼ teaspoon of the salt until crumbly; set aside.

2. In a large bowl, sprinkle the arrowroot evenly over the pears and toss until thoroughly coated. Fold in the remaining 2 tablespoons Sucanat and ½ teaspoon salt, the jam, dried apricots, lemon juice, almond extract, and vanilla extract until well mixed.

3. Fill the baking dish with the fruit mixture and sprinkle evenly with the crumble mixture. Bake for 30 to 35 minutes, until browned and bubbling.

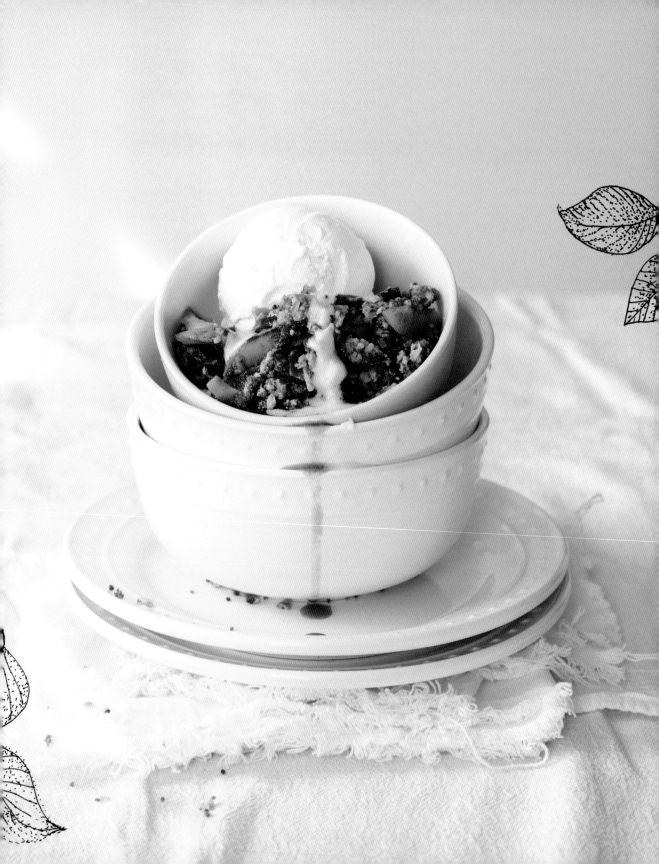

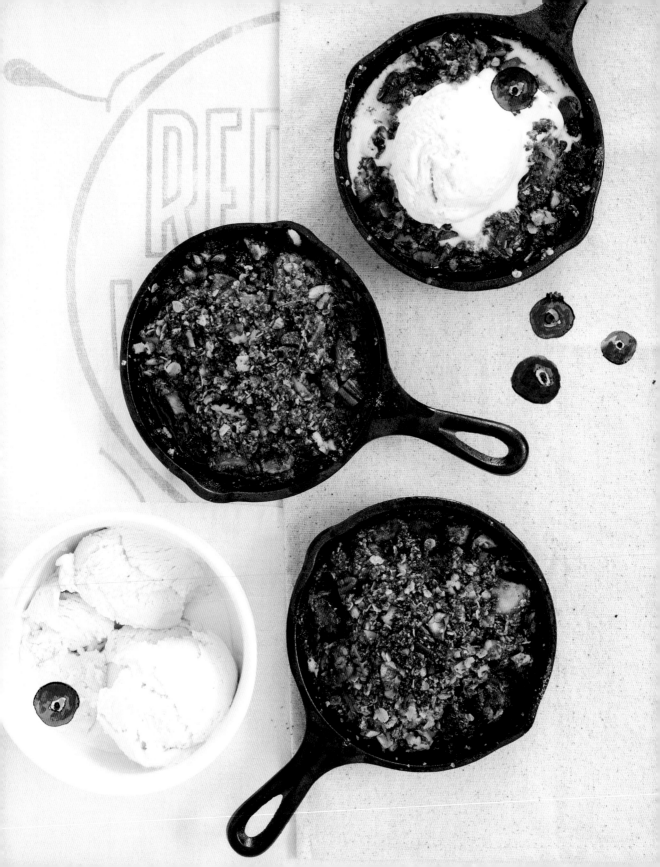

Cast-Iron Cranberry-Apple Crisp

Tart pops of cranberry combined with a sweet and fragrant mix of apples and spice—cooked to golden brown perfection in a no-fuss cast-iron skillet (or multiple minis). If you know what's good for you, serve it warm with coconut cream or vanilla Nice Cream (page 279).

SERVES 6+

⅓ cup (80 ml) unrefined coconut oil, plus more for greasing (solid or liquid)

¾ cup (80 g) oat flour

½ cup (40 g) rolled oats

¼ cup (25 g) raw, unsalted pecans, chopped finely

¼ cup (25 g) raw, unsalted walnuts, chopped finely

¾ cup (150 g) coconut sugar

¾ teaspoon sea salt

2 teaspoons arrowroot starch/flour

3 red apples (Pink Lady, Braeburn, or Fuji), diced (about 6 cups/750 g)

½ cup (50 g) fresh cranberries

3 tablespoons fresh orange juice

3 teaspoons peeled, grated fresh ginger—almost a pulp

1 teaspoon grated orange zest

1 teaspoon ground cinnamon

¼ teaspoon fresh ground nutmeg

1. Preheat the oven to 375°F (190°C) and lightly grease a 10- to 12-inch cast-iron skillet (or six 5-inch/12.5 cm minis) with coconut oil and set aside. In a medium bowl, use a fork to combine the oat flour, oats, oil, pecans, walnuts, ¼ cup (50 g) of the sugar, and ¼ teaspoon of the salt until well combined; set aside this crumble mixture.

2. In a large bowl, sprinkle the arrowroot evenly over the apples and cranberries and toss until thoroughly coated. Add the remaining ½ cup (100 g) sugar, the orange juice, ginger, zest, cinnamon, nutmeg, and remaining ½ teaspoon salt until well mixed.

3. Fill the skillet (or minis) with the fruit mixture and top evenly with the crumble mixture. Bake for 30 to 35 minutes, until browned and bubbling.

Resources

YumUniverse.com

Meal plans, books, recipes, and inspiration.

Instagram: YumUniverse
Snapchat: YumUniverse
Facebook: YumUniverse
Twitter: YumUniverse
Youtube: YumUniverse
Vimeo: YumUniverse
Pinterest: HeatherCrosby

GlutenFreeBakingAcademy.com

With Heather as your guide, learn to make the game-changing, gluten-free, gum-free baked goods you see in this book like toast, buns, and tortillas.

Bonus Resources for Book Owners

There isn't enough room to list all of the shopping tips, ingredient recs, websites, cookbooks, how-tos, helpful podcasts, and other inspiration I'd like to share with you so I've created a special place where *Pantry to Plate* book owners can get it all:

yumuniverse.com/pantry-to-plate-extras

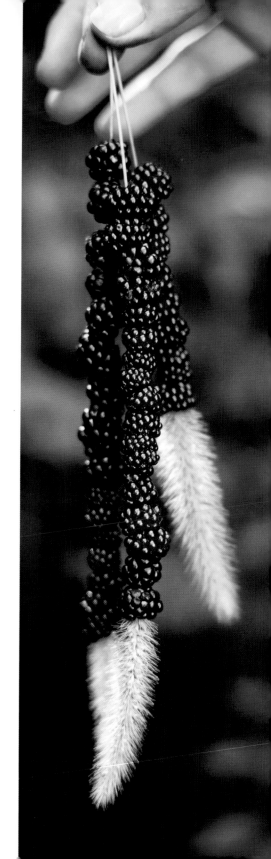

Measurements & Conversions

Psyllium Husk

1 tablespoon whole
psyllium husk =
2½ teaspoons ground

Ginger

*Fresh is recommended
over dried, but in a pinch:*

1 tablespoon peeled,
grated fresh ginger =
½ teaspoon ground

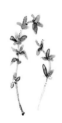

Fresh Herbs,
Dry Herbs

*Fresh is recommended
over dried, but in a pinch:*

1 tablespoon fresh herbs =
1 teaspoon dried

Garlic

*Fresh is recommended
over dried, but in a pinch:*

1 clove =
⅛ teaspoon garlic powder =
½ teaspoon garlic flakes

Onion

*Fresh is recommended
over dried, but in a pinch:*

1 small onion =
1 teaspoon onion powder =
1 tablespoon dried
onion flakes

Dry Grains/
Cooked Grains

A general rule of thumb:

1 cup dry grains + 2½ cups
(600 ml) water/stock =
2+ cups cooked

Dry Beans &
Legumes/
Cooked Beans &
Legumes

A general rule of thumb:

1 cup dry beans or
legumes + 3 to 4 cups
(720 to 960 ml) water/
stock = 3+ cups cooked

Metric Conversions

Vegetables, raw — 1 cup

Artichokes, marinated	260 g
Arugula	20 g
Asparagus, chopped	135 g
Avocado, chopped	150 g
Beet greens, chopped	40 g
Beets, chopped	135 g
Bell pepper (any kind), chopped	150 g
Bok choy, chopped	70 g
Broccoli, chopped	90 g
Brussels sprouts	90 g
Butternut squash, chopped	140 g
Cabbage, chopped	70 g
Capers	140 g
Carrots, chopped	130 g
Cauliflower, chopped	105 g
Celery, chopped	100 g
Chard, packed	35 g
Chicories (endive, frisée, radicchio)	50 g
Cucumber, chopped	135 g
Daikon radish, chopped	115 g
Eggplant, chopped	80 g
Fennel bulb, sliced	85 g
Flowers, edible	20 g
Fresh herbs, chopped	40 g
Green beans, chopped	200 g
Green peas	145 g
Jicama, chopped	120 g
Kale, chopped	15 g
Kohlrabi, chopped	135 g
Leeks, chopped	90 g
Lettuce, chopped	55 g
Mushrooms, chopped	70 g
Olives, pitted	180 g
Onion (any kind), chopped	160 g
Parsnips, chopped	135 g
Potatoes, chopped	150 g
Pumpkin, chopped	115 g
Pumpkin purée	245 g
Radishes, sliced	115 g
Rutabaga, chopped	140 g
Scallions, chopped	100 g
Shallot, chopped	160 g
Spinach	30 g
Summer squash, sliced	115 g
Sweet corn kernels	145 g
Sweet potatoes, chopped	135 g
Tomatoes, chopped	180 g
Tomatoes, sun-dried	110 g
Turnips, chopped	130 g
Watercress, chopped	35 g
Winter squash, chopped	115 g
Yuca (cassava), chopped	205 g
Zucchini, chopped	125 g

Fruits — 1 cup

Apples, chopped	125 g
Apples, dried	85 g
Applesauce	245 g
Apricots, dried	130 g
Banana, mashed	225 g
Banana, sliced	150 g
Blackberries	145 g
Blueberries	145 g
Cherries, pitted	155 g
Cherries, dried	160 g
Coconut, dried (shredded or flaked)	85 g
Coconut, fresh, shredded	80 g
Cranberries, dried	160 g
Crystallized ginger, chopped	160 g
Dates, pitted	150 g
Figs, dried	150 g
Mango, chopped	165 g
Mango, dried	115 g
Melon, chopped	160 g
Nectarines, sliced	145 g
Peaches, sliced	155 g
Pears, chopped	160 g
Pineapple, chopped	165 g
Pineapple, dried	160 g
Plums, sliced	165 g
Prunes, dried	175 g
Raisins	165 g
Raspberries	125 g
Strawberries, whole	145 g

Flours | 1 cup

Blanched almond flour	110 g
Brown rice flour	160 g
Buckwheat flour	120 g
Garbanzo bean flour	120 g
Gluten-free all-purpose flour	150 g
Hazelnut flour/meal	110 g
Oat flour	105 g
Sorghum flour	120 g
Teff flour	165 g

Grains | 1 cup

Amaranth	195 g
Amaranth, cooked	245 g
Brown rice	190 g
Brown rice, cooked	195 g
Brown rice flakes	100 g
Hulled buckwheat groats	165 g
Hulled buckwheat groats, cooked	170 g
Millet	200 g
Millet, cooked	175 g
Oats, rolled	80 g
Oats, steel cut	175 g
Polenta	140 g
Polenta, cooked	235 g
Puffed grains (rice, millet)	15 g
Quinoa	170 g
Quinoa, cooked	185 g
Quinoa flakes	100 g
Rice, cooked	190 g
Teff, cooked	250 g

Legumes | 1 cup

Beans	200 g
Beans, cooked	180 g
Chickpeas	200 g
Chickpeas, cooked	165 g
Lentils	190 g
Lentils, cooked	200 g

Nuts & Seeds | 1 cup

Almonds	145 g
Brazil nuts	135 g
Cashews	135 g
Chia seeds	190 g
Flaxseeds	170 g
Hazelnuts	135 g
Hemp seeds	160 g
Macadamia nuts	135 g
Nuts & seeds, mixed	140 g
Pecan halves	100 g
Pepitas (pumpkin seeds)	130 g
Pine nuts	135 g
Poppy seeds	140 g
Sesame seeds	140 g
Sunflower seeds	140 g
Walnut halves	100 g

Other | 1 cup

Chocolate, dairy-free, chips or chopped	180 g
Coconut cream (from top of chilled can of coconut milk)	220 g
Cream cheese, dairy-free	240 g
Croutons	30 g
Fruit jam, purée, or compote	320 g
Granola	120 g
Hummus	240 g
Kimchi	150 g
Mayonnaise, vegan	225 g
Molasses	335 g
Nutritional yeast	60 g
Sweetener (Sucanat, rapadura, coconut sugar)	200 g
Yogurt, dairy-free	225 g

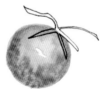

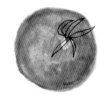

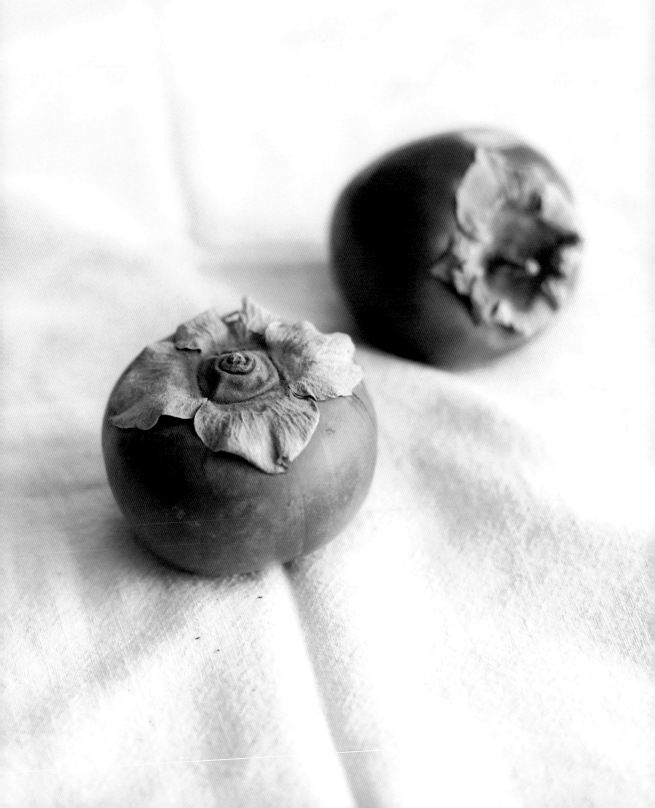

Acknowledgments

Thank you to Matthew Lore, Sarah Smith, Jennifer Hergenroeder, Jeanne Tao, and the team at The Experiment for the opportunity to create this book. Thank you to my editor, Joan Strasbaugh, for your availability and guidance. Thank you to my agent, Linda Konner, for having my back from the very beginning.

Thank you to the YumUniverse community for inspiring me every day. I'm lucky that you spend your time with me. And sweet recipe testers: your honesty and invaluable feedback no doubt made this book better.

Jessica Murnane, thank you for your inspiring podcast, which kept me company on countless clear-my-head walks along the Potomac River, for your generosity of spirit, friendship, feedback, and kindness—it was so special to be writing book babies at the same time.

Kathy Beymer, my dear friend, you were an incredible support during the entire creation of this book. Thank you for your time, your shoulder, and your thoughtful, wise, and generous insights all these years.

Bernardine Somers, where would I be without our walks, talks, and your willingness to come over and enthusiastically try whatever I cooked up each week? Thank you for being such a good friend to me and the book.

Marta Sasinowska, tackle-hug thanks for your talents, for always being there with great taste, laughs, adventure stories, and feedback. And *Dziekuję* to Mama and Papa Sasinowscy, and thank you to Lori Robertson and Chris Crawford for making these pages more beautiful with images from your no-doubt-love-filled gardens.

Pang Tubhirun, thank you for your talent, time, and expertise. And for pointing out the one simple thing I need to do most when taking a photo.

Thanks to my friends and family for your infinite enthusiasm.

And my M. You make me laugh, you ground me, and every time you walk in the room, I fall for you even more. Thanks for taking on book two with me.

Cook-by-Ingredient Index

Have a lot of tomatoes from the garden? Wondering what to make with quinoa? Start with the ingredient—let this quick list inspire a variety delicious eats.

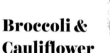

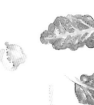
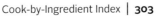

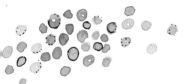

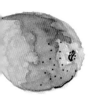
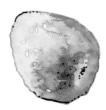
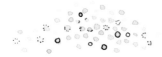

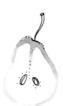
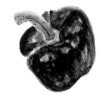
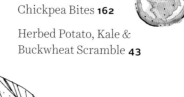

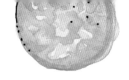
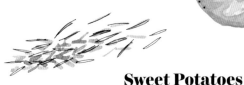

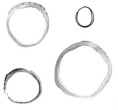

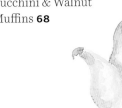
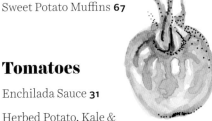
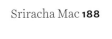

Recipe Index

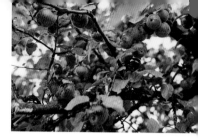

Note: Page numbers in *italics* indicate a photograph.

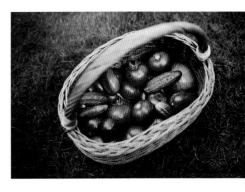

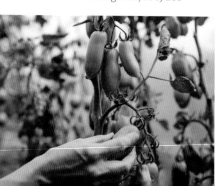

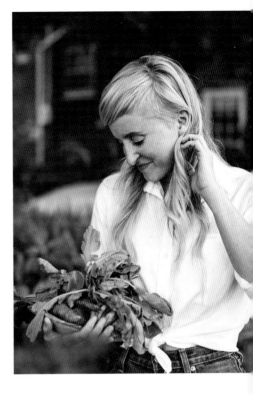

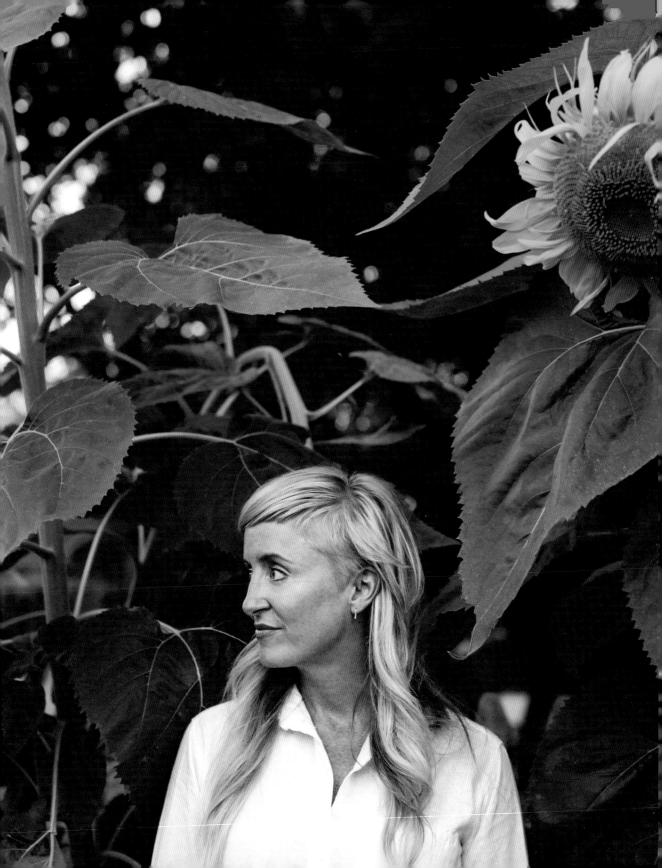

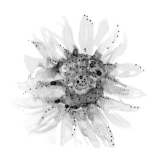

About the Author

Heather Crosby is a former veggie phobe turned veggie lover who lives in a historic small town in West Virginia. Like many folks who find their way to clean eating, she became accountable for her health because she had to, and she continues to work on it every day.

Heather has a plant-based certification from the T. Colin Campbell Center for Nutrition Studies. And she's a big believer that everyone comes to the table with varied habits, beliefs, traditions, and dietary needs, and these layers change and evolve over a lifetime.

She's not interested in being the food police, or telling you how to eat. She's interested in connecting with other health-minded peeps, sharing resources, and providing inspiration for anyone who wants to simply eat more plants and not compromise the "flavor" in their life to do so.

She's a recipe developer and wellness advocate who approaches food through a creative, plant-inspired lens—thinking outside of the box a bit to create shareable, comforting recipes that surprise skeptics and simply make the heart and taste buds happy.

Heather is the creator of GlutenFreeBakingAcademy.com, author of *YumUniverse: Infinite Possibilities for a Gluten-Free, Plant-Powerful, Whole-Food Lifestyle,* and the founder of YumUniverse.com, where over 500 free recipes and helpful resources like meal plans for whole-food, plant-powerful cooking can be discovered.

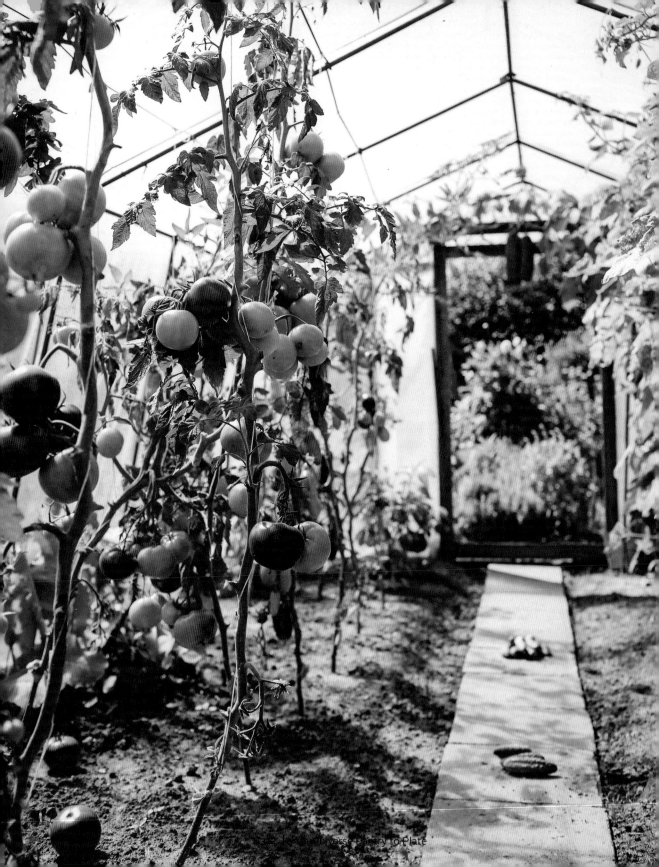